CNA Study Guide

Nurse Assistant Complete Test Prep

Volume One

_____

Jane John-Nwankwo   RN, MSN

CNA Study Guide:
Nurse Assistant Complete Test Prep
Volume One

ISBN-13: 978-1500638702

ISBN-10: 1500638706

Printed in the United States of America.

Have you bought these books?

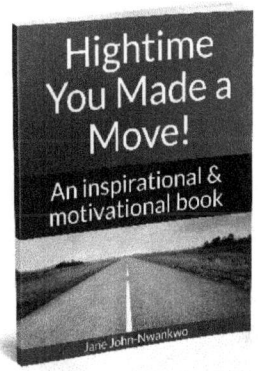

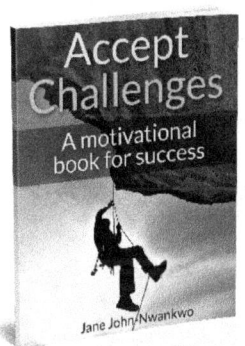

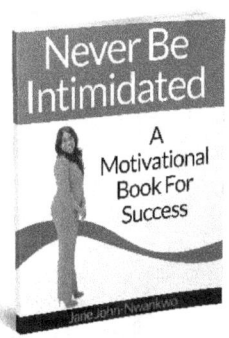

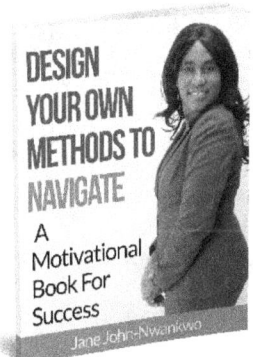

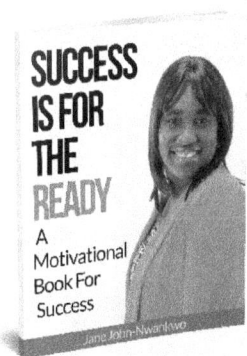

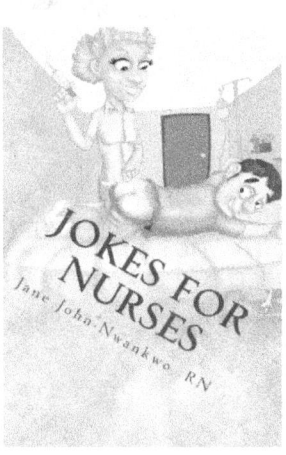

Buy these books at www.bestamericanhealthed.com/resources.html

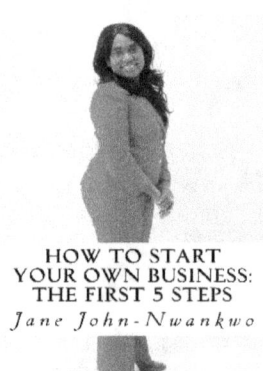

HOW TO START
YOUR OWN BUSINESS:
THE FIRST 5 STEPS
Jane John-Nwankwo

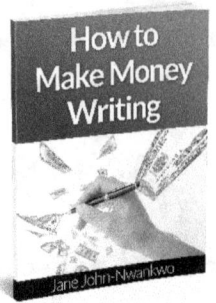

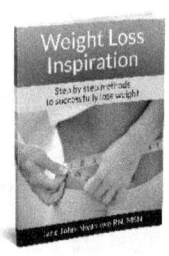

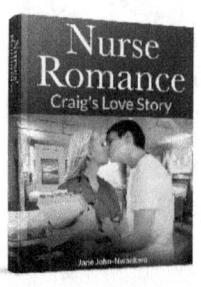

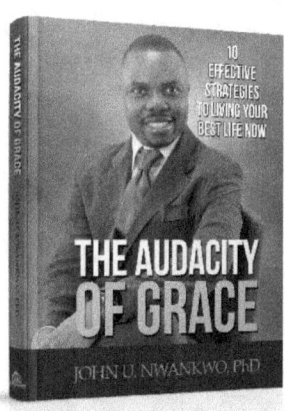

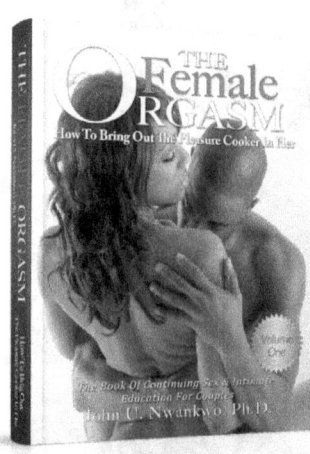

Buy these books at www.bestamericanhealthed.com/resources.html

Dedication

To one of the best CNA instructors: Erika Patterson

OTHER TITLES FROM THE SAME AUTHOR:

1. Work At Home Jobs For Nurses & Other Healthcare Professionals

2. Nurses' Romance Series

3. Hightime you made a move! An inspirational and motivational book

4. Patient Care Technician Exam Review Questions: PCT Test Prep

5. Design Your Own Methods To Navigate

6. EKG Technician Study Guide

7. BLS for Healthcare Providers Student Manual

8. Phlebotomy Test Prep Vol 1, 2, & 3

9. The Home Health Aide Textbook

10. Accept Challenges

And Many More Books

Visit www.healthcarepracticetest.com

www.janejohn-nwankwo.com

www.bookaspeakernow.com

In this book, you will review:

The Medical History

Vital Signs

Patient Care Positions

Safety in the Healthcare Environment

Cardio-pulmonary Resuscitation

Infection Control

More than 150 review questions

Section One

General Information For The Nurse Assistants

Nurse Assistants, also known as nursing aides, geriatric aides, unlicensed assistive personnel, or hospital attendants, perform routine tasks under the supervision of nursing and medical staff. They answer patients' call lights, deliver messages, serve meals, make beds, and help patients eat, dress, and bathe. CNAs also may provide skin care to patients; take their temperatures, pulse rate, respiration rate, and blood pressure; and help patients get in and out of bed and walk. They also may escort patients to operating and examining rooms, keep patients' rooms neat, set up equipment, store and move supplies, or assist with some procedures. They observe patients' physical, mental, and emotional conditions and report any change to the nursing or medical staff.

CNAs help care for physically or mentally ill, injured, disabled, or infirm individuals confined to hospitals, nursing care facilities, and mental health settings. Home health aides' duties are similar, but they work in patients' homes or residential care facilities.

This is usually an entry level for individuals who wish to become nurses in the future. Students are taught principles of infection control, communication techniques, and the skills to safely care for people. These skills include bathing, dressing, assisting to eat, grooming, toileting, lifting and moving while using proper body mechanics.

Upon completion of the nurse assistant training course, students will be able to:

Technical Skills

- Demonstrate awareness of industry standards.

- Define Title 22 regulations regarding the rights of patients.

- Follow hospital safety rules; discuss the role of a nurse assistant in an emergency.

- Practice proper use of body mechanics and positioning techniques using devises for patient comfort and safety.

- Practice centigrade and Fahrenheit conversions for weight, length and liquid volume.

- Demonstrate ability to bathe, dress, and perform personal hygiene tasks for patients.

- Demonstrate ability to collect specimens, remove urinary catheters, apply dressings and make beds.

- Take temperature, pulse and respiration; take accurate blood pressure; document findings.

- Distinguish between types of diet therapies; serve and feed patients.

- Recognize signs and symptoms of distress; react and intervene appropriately.

- Demonstrate ability to care for patients with neurological disorders and aged residents.

- Assist patient with rehabilitative processes and with activities of daily living.

Personal and Professional Skills

- Discuss disinfection and sterilization, hazardous waste disposal, and standard precautions.

- Demonstrate effective patient care documentation.

- Discuss stages of dying and related care; interaction with families; and post-mortem care.

- Demonstrate appropriate work ethics and professional demeanor as demanded by the industry.

- Demonstrate the ability to work independently or as a member of a team.

- Listen attentively, follow directions and effectively relay directions to others.

Career Planning Skills

- Research career opportunities; establish educational and career goals related to the health care industry.

- Research employment opportunities; prepare a resume; prepare for an interview.

When preparing to sit for the state exam as a CNA, I would highly recommend my

books: CNA Exam Prep Volume One and Two, available at

www.bestamericanhealthed.com/resources.html

WORKING CONDITIONS

Most full-time nurse assistants work about 40 hours a week. However, since some

patients need care 24 hours a day, some CNAs work evenings, nights, weekends, and

holidays. Many work part time. Nurse Assistants spend many hours standing and

walking, and they often face heavy workloads. Because they may have to move patients

in and out of bed or help them stand or walk, aides must guard against back injury. CNAs

also may face hazards from minor infections and major diseases, such as hepatitis, but

can avoid infections by following proper procedures.

CNAs often have unpleasant duties, such as emptying bedpans and changing soiled bed

linens. The patients they care for may be disoriented, irritable, or uncooperative. While

their work can be emotionally demanding, many CNAs gain satisfaction from assisting

those in need.

JOB OUTLOOK

Numerous job openings for patient care technicians will arise from a combination of fast

employment growth and high replacement needs. High replacement needs in this large occupation reflect modest entry requirements, low pay, high physical and emotional demands, and lack of opportunities for advancement. For these same reasons, many people are unwilling to perform the kind of work required by the occupation. Therefore, persons who are interested in, and suited for, this work should have excellent job opportunities.

Overall employment of patient care technicians is projected to grow for all occupations through the year 2020, although individual occupational growth rates will vary. Employment of CNAs is expected to grow the fastest, as a result of both growing demand for home healthcare services from an aging population and efforts to contain healthcare costs by moving patients out of hospitals and nursing care facilities as quickly as possible. Consumer preference for care in the home and improvements in medical technologies for in-home treatment also will contribute to faster-than-average employment growth for CNAs and HHAs.

The Medical History

Parts of the patient's medical history are:

-Chief complaint (CC): the reason why the patient came to see the physician.

- History of present illness (HPI): this is an explanation of the chief complaint to determine the onset of the illness; associated symptoms; what the patient has done to treat the condition, etc.

-Past, Family and Social History (PFSH):

- Past medical history: includes all health problems, major illnesses, surgeries the patient has had, current medications complete with reasons for taking them, and allergies.

- Family history: summary of health problems of siblings, parents, and other blood relatives that could alert the physician to hereditary and/or familial diseases.

-Social history: includes marital status, occupation, educational attainment, hobbies, use of alcohol, tobacco, drugs, and lifestyles.

-Review of Systems - this is an orderly and systematic check of each organ and system of the body by questions. Both positive and pertinent negative findings are documented. The ROS, in conjunction with the physical examination, helps elicit information that is essential to the diagnosis of patient's condition.

Vital Signs

Reflect the functions of three body processes necessary for life:

Body temperature

Respiration

Heart function

The four vital signs of body function are:

Temperature

Pulse

Respiration

Blood pressure

Temperature

Body temperature is a balance between heat production and heat loss in conjunction with each other, maintained and regulated by the hypothalamus.

Thermometers are used to measure temperature using the Fahrenheit and Centigrade or Celsius scale. Temperature sites are the following: mouth, rectum, ear (tympanic membrane), and the axilla (underarm). The normal ranges for each site are:

Site	Normal Range
Rectal	98.6F to 100.6F (37.0C to 38.1C)
Oral	97.6F to 99.6F (36.5C to 37.5C)
Axillary	96.6F to 98.6F (35.9C to 37.0C)
Tympanic Membrane	98.6F (37C)

Some terms used to describe body temperature are:

Febrile – presence of fever

Afebrile – absence of fever

Fever – elevated body temperature beyond normal range. Types of fever are:

Intermittent: fluctuating fever that returns to or below baseline then rises again.

Remittent: fluctuating fever that remains elevated; it does not return to baseline temperature.

Continuous: a fever that remains constant above the baseline; it does not fluctuate.

Oral temperature is the most common method of measurement; however, it is not taken from   the   following   patients:

- infants and children less than six years old

- patients who has had surgery or facial, neck, nose, or mouth injury

- those receiving oxygen

- those with nasogastric tubes

- patients with convulsive seizure

- hemiplegic patients

- patients with altered mental status

Wait for 30 minutes to take the oral temperature in patients who have just finished eating, drinking, or smoking. When taking the temperature, leave the thermometer in the patient's mouth for 3-5 minutes or as required by agency policy.

Rectal temperature is taken when oral temperature is not feasible. However, it is not taken from the following patients:

- patients with heart disease

- patients with rectal disease or disorder or has had rectal surgery

- patients with diarrhea

It is taken with the patient in a side-lying position and the thermometer and the patient's hip is held throughout the procedure so the thermometer is not lost in the rectum or broken.

Axillary temperature is the least accurate and is taken only when no other temperature site can be used. The axilla, (the underarm) should be clean and dry and the thermometer should be held in place for 5-10 minutes or as required by the facility policy.

Tympanic temperature is useful for children and confused patients because of the speed of operation of the tympanic thermometer. A covered probe is gently inserted into the ear canal and temperature is measured within seconds (1–3 seconds). It is not used if the patient has an ear disorder or ear drainage.

Pulse

The normal adult pulse rate ranges between 60 and 100 beats per minute. The site most commonly used for taking pulse is the radial artery found in the wrist on the same side as the thumb. It is felt with the first two or three fingers (never with the thumb) and usually taken for 30 seconds multiplied by two to get the rate per minute. If the rate is unusually fast or slow, however, count it for 60 seconds.

The apical pulse is a more accurate measurement of the heart rate and it is taken over the apex of the heart by auscultation using the stethoscope. It is used for patients with irregular heart rate and for infants and small children.

Respiration

When measuring respiration, respiratory characteristics such as rate, rhythm, and depth are taken into account. Rate is the number of respirations per minute. The normal range for adults is 12 to 20 per minute. One inspiration (inhale) and one expiration (exhale) counts as one respiration. It is counted for 30 seconds multiplied by two or for a full minute.

Some rate abnormalities are the following:

Apnea – this is a temporary complete absence of breathing which may be a result of a reduction in the stimuli to the respiratory centers of the brain.

Tachypnea – this is a respiration rate of greater than 40/min. It is transient in the newborn and maybe caused by the hysteria in the adult.

Bradypnea – decrease in numbers of respirations. This occurs during sleep. It may also be   due   to   certain   diseases. Respiratory rhythm refers to the pattern of breathing. It can vary with age: infants have an irregular rhythm while adults have regular.

Some abnormalities in the rhythm are the following:

Cheyne-Stokes – this is a regular pattern of irregular breathing rate.

Orthopnea – this is difficulty or inability to breath unless in an upright position.

Depth of respiration refers to the amount of air that is inspired and expired during each respiration. Some abnormalities in the depth of respirations are the following:

Hypoventilation: state in which reduced amount of air enters the lungs resulting in decreased oxygen level and increased carbon dioxide level in blood. It can be due to breathing that is too shallow, or too slow, or to diminished lung function.

Hyperpnea: abnormal increase in the depth and rate of breathing.

Hyperventilation: state in which there is an increased amount of air entering the lungs.

Blood Pressure

This is the measurement of the amount of force exerted by the blood on the peripheral arterial walls and is expressed in millimeters (mm) of mercury (Hg). The measurement consist of two components: the highest (systole) and lowest (diastole) amount of pressure exerted during the cardiac cycle.

A stethoscope and sphygmomanometer of either aneroid or mercury type are used. The size of the cuff of the sphygmomanometer will depend on the circumference of the limb and not the age of the patient. The width of the inflatable bag within the cuff should be about 40% of this circumference – 12 cm to 14 cm in an average adult. The length of the bag should be about 80% of this circumference – almost long enough to encircle the arm. Cuffs that are too short or narrow may give falsely high readings, e.g. a regular cuff on an obese arm may lead to a false diagnosis of hypertension.

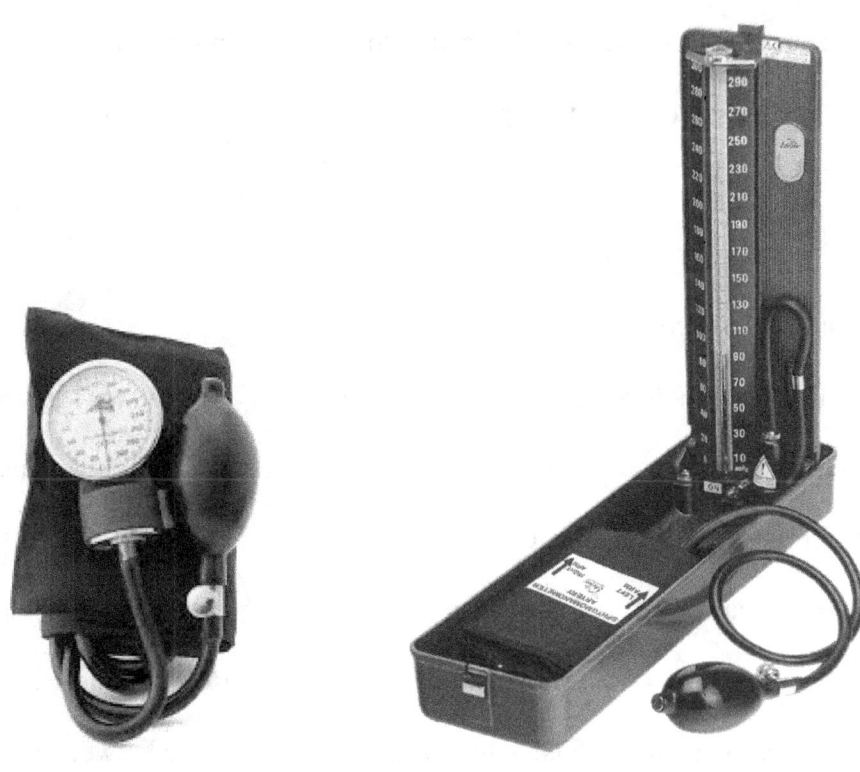

The inflatable bag is centered over the brachial artery with the lower border about 2.5cm above the antecubital crease. The cuff is positioned at heart level. If the brachial artery is far below the heart level the blood pressure will appear falsely high. If the brachial artery is far above heart level, blood pressure will appear falsely low.

Blood pressure is taken by determining first the palpatory systolic pressure over the brachial artery. Then with the bell of the stethoscope over the brachial artery, the cuff is inflated again to about 30 mm Hg above the palpatory systolic pressure and deflated slowly, allowing the pressure to drop at a rate of about 2 to 3 mmHg per second. Note the level at which you hear the sounds of at least two consecutive beats. This is the systolic pressure. Continue to lower the pressure slowly until the sounds become muffled and then disappear. Then deflate the cuff rapidly to zero. The disappearance point, which is usually only a few mmHg below the muffling point, marks the generally accepted diastolic pressure. Both the systolic and diastolic pressure levels are read the nearest 2 mmHg.

Common errors in blood pressure measurements:

Improper cuff size. Cuffs that are too short or narrow may give falsely high readings. Using a regular cuff on an obese arm may lead to a false diagnosis of hypertension. For an obese arm, select a cuff with a larger than standard bag.

The arm is not at heart level. If the brachial artery is much below the heart level, the blood pressure will appear falsely high. Conversely, if the artery is much above heart level, blood pressure will appear falsely low. A 13.6 cm difference between arterial and cardiac levels produces a blood pressure error of 10mmHg.

Cuff is not completely deflated before use. Deflation of the cuff is faster than 2-3 mmHg per second. Rapid deflation will lead to underestimation of the systolic and overestimation of the diastolic

pressure.

The cuff is re-inflated during the procedure without allowing the arm to rest for 1-2 minute between readings. Repetitive inflation of the cuff can result in venous congestion, which could make the sound less audible producing artifactually low systolic and high diastolic pressure.

Improper cuff placement.

Defective equipment. A bag that balloons outside the cuff leads to falsely high readings.

Anthropometric Measurements

The term anthropometric refers to comparative measurements of the body. They are used as indicators of the state of health and well-being of the patient and are often included in the initial measurement of vital signs. Anthropometric measurements require precise measuring techniques to be valid.

Length, height, weight, weight-for-length, and head circumference (length is used in infants and toddlers, rather than height, because they are unable to stand) are used to assess growth and development in infants, children and adolescents. Individual measurements are usually compared to reference standards on a growth chart.

Height, weight, body mass index (BMI), waist-to-hip ratio, and percentage of body fat are the measurements used for adults. These measures are then compared to reference standards to assess weight status and the risk for various diseases.

Patient Care Positions

Positioning a Patient for Examination or Treatment

When performing an examination, treatment, tests or to obtain specimens, patients are put in special positions.

The Horizontal Recumbent Position is used for most physical examinations. The patient lies on his/her back with legs extended. Arms may be above the head, alongside the body or folded on the chest.

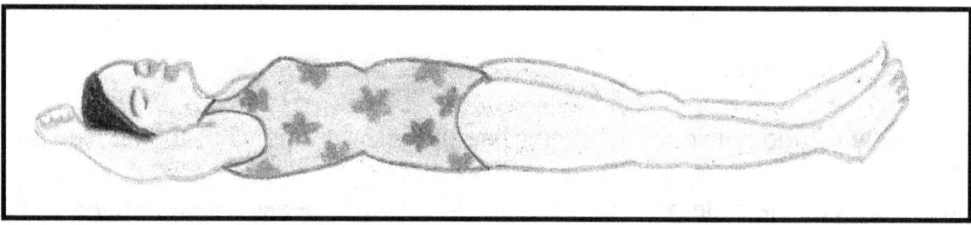

Figure 1-1. Horizontal recumbent position.

The Dorsal Recumbent Position is when the patient is on his/her back with knees flexed and soles of the feet flat on the bed. The PCT will need to fold a sheet once across the chest and fold a second sheet crosswise over the thighs and legs so that genital area is easily exposed.

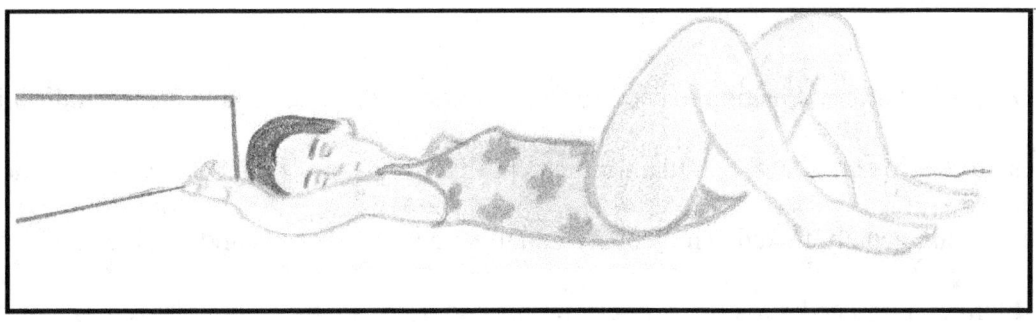

Figure 1-2. Dorsal recumbent position

The Fowler's Position is used to promote drainage or to ease breathing. A sitting or semi-sitting position where the back of the examination table is elevated to either 45 degrees (Semi-Fowler's) or 90 degrees (High- Fowler's). The knees maybe raised slightly by placing a pillow underneath, but usually the legs rest flat on the table. . The patient may need a foot support. This position is usually used for patients with cardiovascular or respiratory problems, and for the examination of the upper body and head.

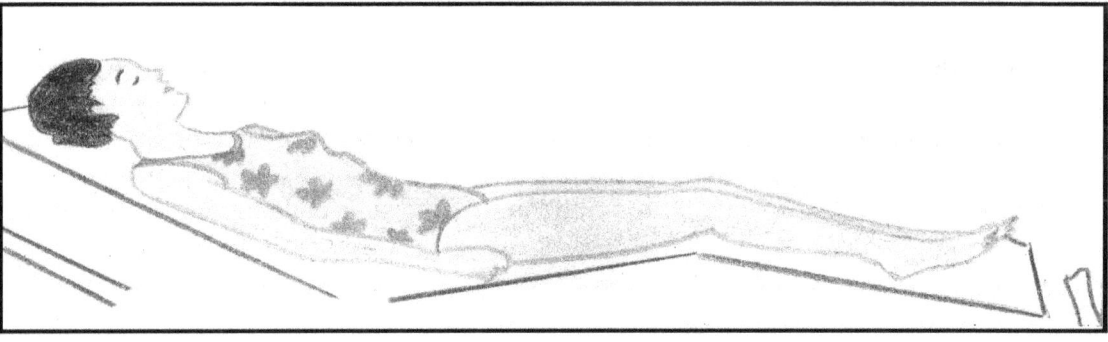

Figure 1-3. Fowler's position.

The Dorsal Lithotomy Position is used for examination of pelvic organs. This position is similar to the dorsal recumbent position, except that the patient's legs are well separated and thighs are acutely flexed. The feet are usually placed in stirrups and a folded sheet or bath blanket is placed crosswise over thighs and legs so that genital area is easily exposed. Keep the patient covered as much as possible.

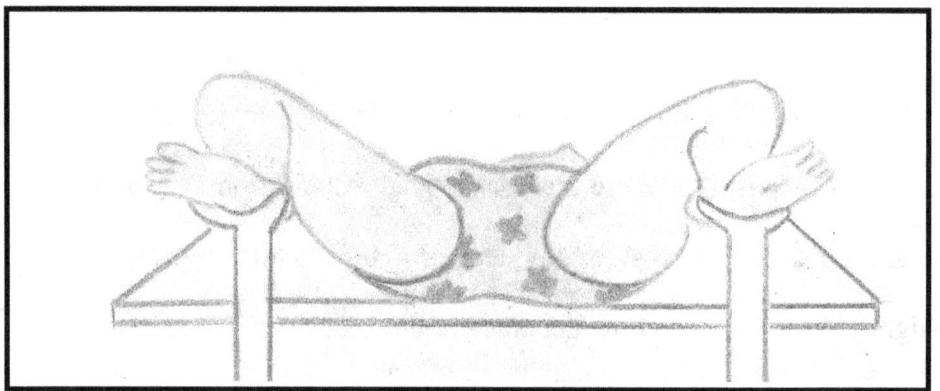

The Prone Position is used to examine the spine and back. The patient lies on his/her abdomen with head turned to one side for comfort, the arms may be above head or alongside the body. Cover with sheet or bath blanket. This position is used in the examination of the posterior aspect of the body, including the back or spine. NOTE: An unconscious patient or one with an abdominal incision or breathing difficulty usually cannot lie in this position.

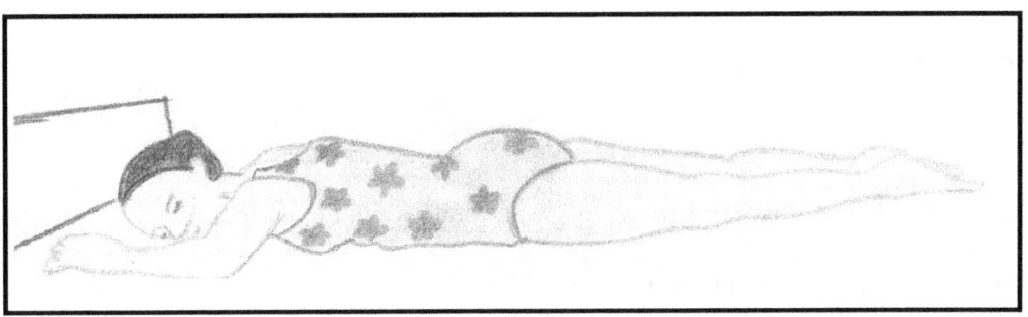

Figure 1-5. Prone position.

The Sim's Position is used for rectal examination. The patient is on his/her left side with the right knee flexed against the abdomen and the left knee slightly flexed. The left arm is behind the body; the right arm is placed comfortably. NOTE: Patient with leg injuries or arthritis usually cannot assume this position.

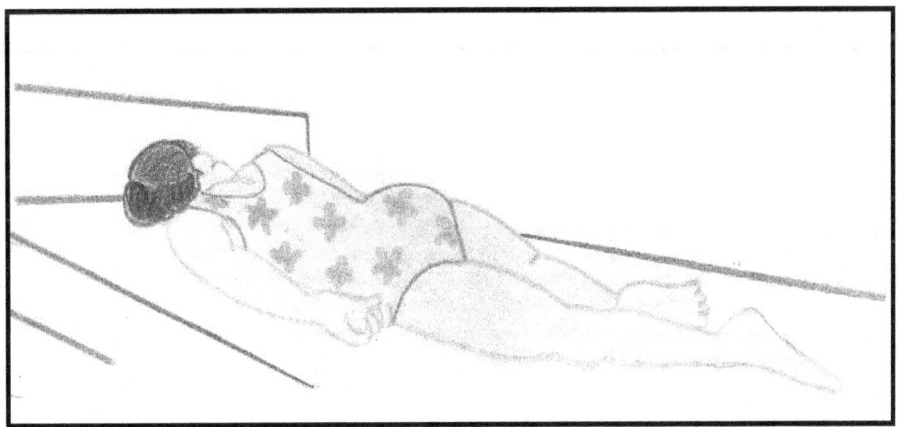

Figure 1-6. Sim's position.

The Knee-Chest Position is used for rectal and vaginal examinations and as treatment to bring the uterus into normal position. The patient is on his/her knees with his/her chest resting on the bed and elbows resting on the bed or arms above head. The head is turned to one side. The thighs are straight and lower legs are flat on the bed. NOTE: Do not leave patient alone; he/she may become dizzy, faint, and fall.

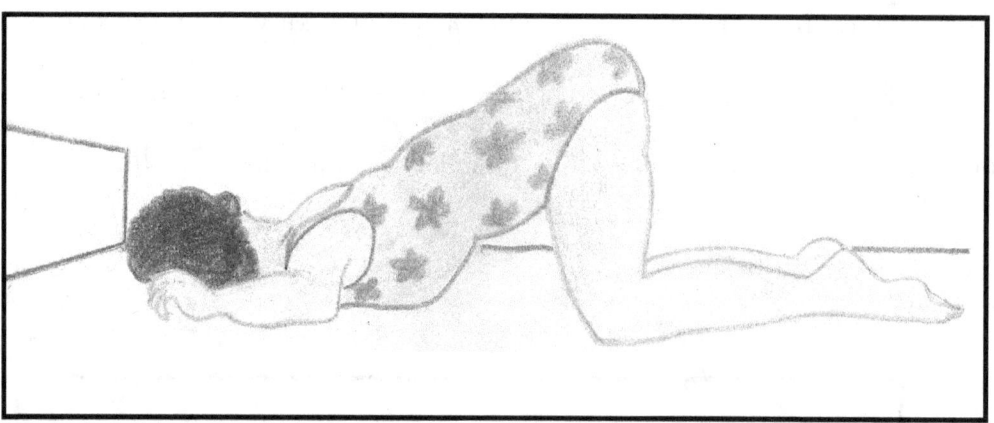

Figure 1-7. Knee-chest position.

Trendelenburg position – The patient is placed flat on the back, face up, the knees flexed and legs hanging off the end of the table, with the legs and feet supported by a footboard. The table is positioned with the head 45 degrees lower than the body. This position is used primarily for surgical procedures of pelvis and abdomen.

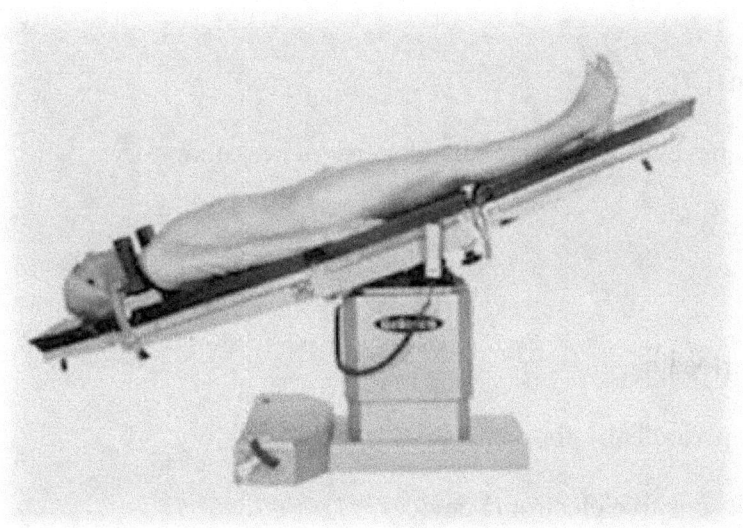

Safety

Safety hazards abound in the healthcare setting, many of which can cause serious injury or disease. The Occupational Safety and Health Administration (OSHA) is responsible for the identification of the various hazards present in the workplace and for the creation of rules and regulations to minimize exposure to such hazards. Employers are mandated to institute measures that will assure safe working conditions and health workers have the obligation to know and follow those measures.

Safety rules are usually based on common sense. Most accidents occur when these rules are neglected, overlooked or ignored. Accidents generally occur when safety is compromised because of haste and secondary shortcuts. These shortcuts can lead to personal injury and equipment damage. When an accident occurs, it must be reported to your supervisor immediately. Trying to cover up the incident can lead to serious, even disastrous results.

Hazards

A. Physical Hazards

Electrical Safety Regulations

Use only ground plugs that have been approved by Underwriters' Laboratory (UL).

Never use extension cords.

Avoid electrical circuit overloading.

Inspect all cords and plugs periodically for damage.

Use a surge protector on all sensitive electronic devices.

Before servicing, UNPLUG the device from the electrical outlet.

Use signs and/or labels to indicate high voltage or electrical hazards.

B. Chemical Hazards

Chemical Safety Regulations

If the skin or eyes come in contact with any chemicals, immediately wash the area with water for at least 5 minutes.

Store flammable or volatile chemicals in a well-ventilated area.

After use, immediately recap all bottles containing toxic substances.

Label all chemicals with the required Material Safety Data Sheet (MDSD) information.

C. Biological Hazards

Biological Safety Regulations

1. Disinfect the laboratory work area before and after each use when dealing with biologicals.

2. Never draw a specimen through a pipette by mouth. This technique is not permitted in the laboratory.

3. Always wear gloves.

4. Sterilize specimens and any other contaminated materials and/or dispose of them through incineration.

5. Wash hands thoroughly before and after every procedure.

Emergency First Aid

The ability to recognize and react quickly to an emergency may be the difference of life or death for the patient. As patients react differently to various situations, it is important for all healthcare professionals to be prepared in an emergency.

External Hemorrhage: controlling the bleeding is most effectively accomplished by elevating the affected part above heart level and applying direct pressure to the wound. Do not attempt to elevate a broken extremity as this could cause further damage. Shock occurs when there is _insufficient return of blood flow to the heart, resulting in inadequate supply of oxygen to all organs and tissues of the body.' Patients experiencing trauma may go into shock and for some patients, seeing their own blood may induce shock.

Common symptoms:

-Pale, cold, clammy skin

-Rapid, weak pulse

- Increased, shallow breathing rate

- Expressionless face/staring eyes.

First Aid for Shock:

-Maintain an open airway for the victim

-Call for assistance

-Keep the victim lying down with the head lower than the rest of the body

-Attempt to control bleeding or cause of shock (if known)

-Keep the victim warm until help arrives

Cardiopulmonary Resuscitation. Most healthcare institutions require their professionals to be certified in CPR. It is important for all professionals to maintain all certifications acquired.

Why do we have to do CPR?

The CPR process is very important to the victim and is composed of several functions. The first function is neutralizing any dangers from the surroundings. The rescuer should ensure any hazards are removed and the victims are well taken care of. The second component is checking the status of the victim by asking questions and if the victim does not respond the rescuer should send for help.

The third component is unblocking the airway and checking for breathing. After checking for breathing, the rescuer is then supposed to start the compressions.

According to Mistovich and Karren (2010) the rescuer should first administer 30 compressions at a rate of 2 compressions per second. All along, the rescuer should make sure the victims are lying on their backs and the head and the chin is lifted. The CPR should be repeated in a cycle of 30 compressions and 2 rescue breaths. If the victim fails to respond to the CPR, an automated external defibrillator should be used. It is very paramount that chest compressions be started immediately, not more than 10 seconds from the time of cardiac arrest. If you don't feel a pulse, or are not sure you feel a pulse, start chest compressions!

According to Mistovich and Karren (2010) chest compressions during CPR generate small but critical amount of blood flow to the heart and brain. Mistovich and Karren (2010) further suggest that the quality of the chest compressions determines the success of the resuscitation. The physiology of chest compressions can be understood using the external; cardiac massage and thoracic pump models. According to Huether and McCance (2004), external cardiac massage compresses the cardiac structures hence forcing the blood to circulate. On the other hand, the thoracic pump model suggests that chest compressions increase the global intra-thoracic pressure. During the CPR process the brain is susceptible to the decreased blood flow and could suffer from irreversible damage within five minutes of absent perfusion. Chest compressions ensure blood circulates to the brains and other susceptible organs such as the myocardium (the muscles of the heart).

The appropriate way to do compressions

Given the importance of the chest compressions, it is important that the rescuer administers them in the right manner. Chest compressions are supposed to be forceful and should be administered on the lower half of the sternum. The victim should be placed in a supine position while the rescuer kneels beside the victim's chest. For compressive force to be effective, the patients should be placed in a firm surface. In addition, interruptions of chest compressions should be avoided and the rescuer should take maximum care not to dislodge lines and tubes. The rescuer should place the dominant hand on the center of the victim's chest. The heel of his or her hands should be positioned in the midline and aligned with the long axis of the sternum. The non-dominant hand should be placed over the dominant one, with the fingers elevated off the patient's ribs. This arrangement ensures the rescuer is able to apply enough

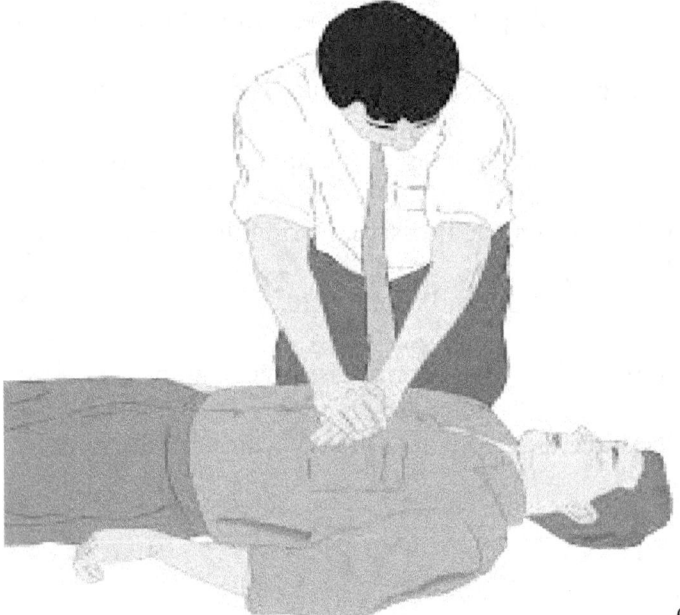

compressive force and to minimize damage of the ribs. The rescuer should avoid applying force over the xiphisternum (tip of the sternum) and the upper abdomen. While applying pressure on the victim's chest, the rescuer should keep his arms straight and extended. The rescuer's shoulders should be positioned vertically above the victim's chest to ensure maximize the effectiveness of the compressive forces. In the article titled, *technique for chest compressions in adult CPR*, Rajab, Conrad, Cohn and Schmitto (2011) suggests that chest compressions should be delivered at a rate of at least 100 per minute and any interruptions should be avoided. In the same article, Rajab, Conrad, Cohn and Schmitto (2011) argue that compression depth should be maintained at 5 cm and the rescuer should allow the victim's chest to recoil completely. In addition, the rescuer should avoid removing his or her hands from the victim's chest, in order to maintain the right compression depth. The rescuer should observe a duty cycle of 50% and the compressor should be rotated every two minutes. Chest compression is terminated after the patient recovers or when the Emergency Response Team arrives to continue ACLS (Advanced Cardio Vascular Life Support).

The BLS Survey

The American Heart Association recommends training of persons to equip them with the necessary skills to save lives. Receiving the CPR training gives the rescuers the ability to perform basic activities such as restoring the blood circulation, clearing the airway, and conducting rescue breathing. One of the major components of the BLS survey is checking the responsiveness of the patient by tapping or shouting. The rescuer is also supposed to determine whether the patient is breathing or not. To determine whether the patient is breathing or not, the rescuer should listen for breath sounds. Alternatively, the rescuer should use the cheeks to feel the flow of air from the patient's breaths. The next key component of the BLS survey is activating the emergency response system and obtaining an automated external defibrillator (AED). According to the acceptable principles, the rescuer is required to activate the Emergency Response System and begin the CPR after establishing that the patient is unresolved and is unable to breathe. Another key step is checking for the carotid pulses. If the patient is unresponsive or if he or she is not breathing well, the rescuer should take not more than 10 seconds in checking for a pulse.

In the absence of a pulse, chest compressions should be administered immediately. As suggested by the 2010s, AHA guidelines for CPR and ECC, the rescuer should adhere to the C-A-B sequence (Compressions-Airway-Breathing). The last component of the BLS survey is defibrillation. A defibrillator or AED is used to check for a shockable rhythm and is normally used in the absence of a pulse.

Pocket masks

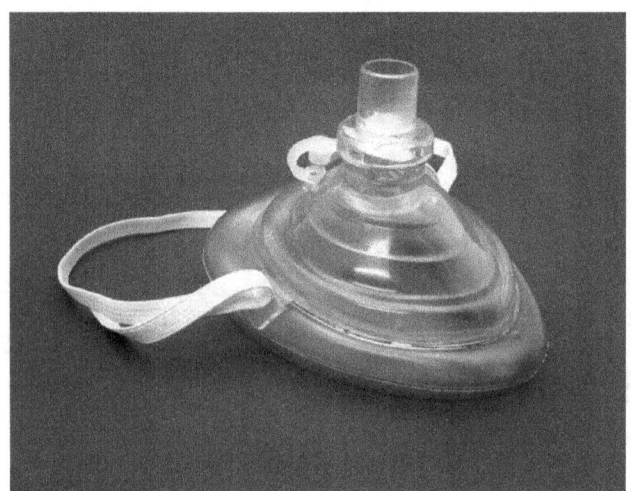

As earlier indicated, mouth-to-mouth resuscitation is the cornerstone of the CPR. However, there is reluctance by the medical professionals to use this type of resuscitation. One of the common reasons given by nurses and the physicians is the fear of contracting diseases and infections. Their observations are supported by a study conducted by Handley (2002) which shows that HIV transmission can occur due to trauma, oral lesions and contact with blood. It is for this reason, that the medical practitioners are advised to carry pocket masks.

Pocket masks are considered to be effective in delivering rescue breaths to the patient during cardiac or respiratory arrest. The pocket masks have a pre-inflated cuff to provide an effective seal around the mouth and the nose. The one-way valve reduce contamination while the in-line filter, filters the air. A pocket mask also has an oxygen inlet port to deliver high-flow oxygen to the patient. The pocket mask is placed on the patient's face with the base of the mask resting between the casualty's chin and the lower lip. The masks are re-usable but the filters and the valve should be discarded after use. According to Handley (2002) the masks are preferred as they create a comfortable distance between the patient and the rescuer. The device also allows the rescuer to observe the chest movements and monitor the patient.

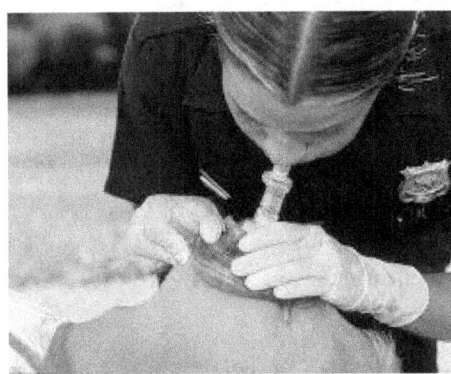

However, while pocket masks are preferred by the medical practitioners, a study conducted by Adelborg et al (2011) indicates that mouth-to-mouth ventilation is superior to mouth-to-pocket masks. In this study, Adelborg et al (2011) used a sample of 60 life guards to perform three sessions of single rescuer CPR. According to Adelborg et al (2011) significantly more ventilation were delivered by the mouth-to-mouth ventilations compared to the mouth-to-pocket masks. But for safety and healthcare reasons, Mouth to mask breathing is resorted to.

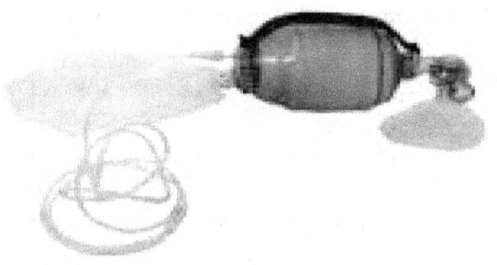

Using the bag mask   This

device provides positive pressure ventilation to the patients, and made up of a bag and

valve combinations. Bag masks have proved to be effective in airway management and

providing patients with enough air. Bag masks come in different sizes and are the

responsibility of the rescuers to choose the most appropriate one. Bag masks are either

attached to the oxygen tank or draw room air.

The device is operated by one whereby the rescuer hold holds the BVM with one

hand, while the other hand compresses the bag delivering the oxygen. The two-person

bag ventilation mask has been shown to be more effective than a singly-operated bag

mask in delivering greater tidal volumes and introducing less air leak.

When using a bag mask, one is required to position himself or herself above the victim's head. The rescuer then places the mask on the victim's head and holds it in position using the E-C device. Once the mask is in place, the rescuer is then required to

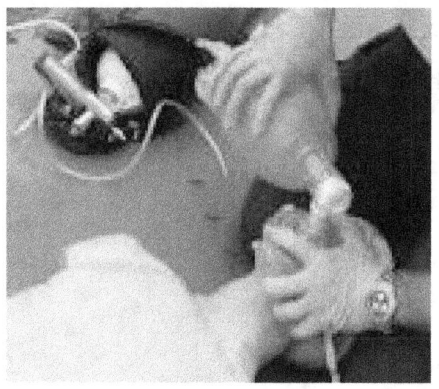

press the bag and watch for the chest rise.

One rescuer CPR and 2 rescuers CPR

There are two basic ways of performing CPR: 1-person CPR and the 2-person CPR. Of the two techniques, the 2-Person CPR is the best, as the victim is able to receive enough air volume and is less tiring. One of the rescuers administers the chest compressions while the other performs the rescue breaths. Alternatively, the two rescuers can switch about every two minutes.

Adult CPR and Child CPR and Infant CPR

In all the patients, the chest compression rate and the sequence is the same: At least 100 compressions per minute. In addition, during the CPR, chest wall recoil should be allowed between compressions and interruption should be limited to less than 10 seconds. The way CPR is administered varies according to the age. The CPR procedure varies among the adults, children and the infants and these differences are shown in the table below.

CPR COMPONENT	ADULTS	CHILDREN	INFANTS
Activating EMS and getting an AED	Call for help and if alone phone EMS immediately	Call for help but if alone, phone EMS after giving 5 cycles of CPR	Call for help but if alone, phone EMS after giving 5 cycles of CPR
COMPRESSION DEPTH	5CM	5CM	4CM
COMPRESSION-VENTILATION RATIO	30:2 1 or 2 rescuers	30:2 Single rescuer 15:2 2 rescuers	30:2 Single rescuer 15:2 2 rescuers
Compression location	Centre of chest	Centre of chest	Just below nipple line on breast bone
Compression method	2hands : heel of 1 hand , other hand on top	1 hand. Or 2 hands if the child is obese. heel of 1 hand , other hand on top	2 fingers: middle and ring or 2 thumbs

While the above shows the differences in CPR entities there are a number of CPR components that are common among the adults, children and the infants. One such component is the type of the response. It is the role of the rescuer to ensure that the environment is safe enough and to establish if the victim is responsive or not. To check for breathing and open the airway, the rescuer is required to tilt the chin and should not take more than five minutes to check for the visual cues such as chest rise. Compression rate in adults, children and the infants should be maintained at a rate of at least 100 compressions per minute while the compression ventilation ration should be held at 30:2. However, for the drowning patients, CPR sequence should start with 2 initiation breaths before chest compressions.

Rescue breathing

Although some of the instructors may not emphasize on rescue breathing, it is considered important in resuscitating the patients. Two breaths are administered for every 30 chest compressions. To breathe air into the patient, the rescuer pinches his or her nose and the closes on the victim's mouth. The rescuer breathes slowly into the victim leading to the rising of the chest. However, a study conducted by Rea et al (2010) insists that there is no need of rescue breathing if the rescuers are not competent enough.

These findings are captured in a randomized trial where 981 of the participants received chest compression only while 960 received chest compression plus rescue breathing. In the end Rea et al (2010) concluded that administering chest compressions alone especially in cancer patients increases the overall survival rate.

Choking for an infant

Choking is very common in small children and is caused by swallowing of huge chunks of food. Some of the other objects that small children choke on include: buttons, carrots and toys. Symptoms of choking in children include high pitched breathing, coughing, color changes and lack of breathing. Choking in infants is treated using back slaps and chest thrusts. To administer the back slaps the baby is supported using one hand, facing upside down. The baby is placed on the laps and the back slaps are then administered using the heel of hand. On the other hand, chest thrusts are administered with the baby facing up. The chest thrusts are applied using two fingers just below the nipple line. So, five chest thrusts, then five back slaps (One cycle). Five cycles must be done. After the fifth cycle, the infant's mouth is opened to see if the object has become visible. If the object has become visible, it is carefully removed. Blind sweeping should never be attempted. If it is not visible, continue the back slaps and chest thrusts until help arrives. If chest becomes unresponsive, commence CPR.

Choking for an adult

Choking in adults occurs when foods and other solids partially or completely block the airway. According to the available statistics, choking is a leading case of home injury death in the United States and adults are at an increased risk of choking due to dental problems and age-related illness.

Other causes of choking include:

- eating too fast

- talking with food in the mouth

-wearing dentures and eating foods with wrong texture.

Symptoms of choking include:

-inability to talk, coughing, fainting and clutching of both hands to the throat, usually referred to the universal choking sign.

In adults and children choking is treated using back blows and abdominal thrusts. Blows and thrusts are administered until the obstruction is dislodged. To apply the blows, the victim is made to bend until he or she is near parallel to the ground. The victim is supported with one arm and then the back blows are administered between the shoulder blades. Alternatively, abdominal thrusts should be given, or chest thrusts if the individual is pregnant.

Conclusion

CPR is an important component of emergency response and leads to significant survival rates of the patients. Despite its success some of the procedures are still archaic and infringe on the rights of the rescuers. For this reason, there is need to address some of the concerns raised by the medical practitioners and conduct extensive research in order to simplify the entire process. The best thing one can do for an unresponsive individual is to start chest compressions before help arrives. THAT SINGLE ACT CAN SAVE THE VICTIM'S LIFE!!!

Infection Control/Chain of Infection

This consists of links, each of which is necessary for the infectious disease to spread. Infection control is based on the fact that the transmission of infectious diseases will be prevented or stopped when any level in the chain is broken or interrupted.

Agent -------------- Mode of transmission ------------ Susceptible host

: :

: :

 portal of exit portal of entry

Agents– are infectious microorganisms that can be classified into groups namely: viruses, bacteria, fungi, and parasites. When infectious diseases are identified according to the specific disease-causing microorganism, the disease may be prevented with the use of anti-infective drugs or infection control practices.

Portal of exit –the method by which an infectious agent leaves its reservoir. Standard Precautions and Transmission-Based Precautions are control measures aimed at preventing the spread of the disease as infectious agents exit the reservoir.

Mode of transmission –specific ways in which microorganisms travel from the reservoir to the susceptible host. There are five main types of mode of transmission:

- Contact : direct and indirect

- Droplet

- Airborne

- Common vehicle

- Vectorborne

Portal of entry – allows the infectious agent access to the susceptible host. Common entry sites are broken skin, mucous membranes, and body systems exposed to the external environment such as the respiratory, gastrointestinal, and reproductive. Methods such as sterile wound care, transmission-based precautions, and aseptic technique limit the transmission of the infectious agents.

Susceptible host – The infectious agent enters a person who is not resistant or immune. Control at this level is directed towards the identification of the patients at risk, treat their underlying condition for susceptibility, or isolate them from the reservoir.

Medical Asepsis

Best defined as —the destruction of pathogenic microorganisms after they leave the body.‖ It also involves environmental hygiene measures such as equipment cleaning and disinfection procedures. Methods of medical asepsis are Standard Precautions and

Transmission-Based Precautions

Disinfection. This procedure used in medical asepsis using various chemicals that can be used to destroy many pathogenic microorganisms. Since chemicals can irritate skin and mucous membranes, they are used only on inanimate objects.

The least expensive and most readily available disinfectant for surfaces such as countertops is a 1:10 solution of household bleach. Boiling water (temperature of 212 F) is considered a form of disinfection, but use of it in today's medical setting is limited to items that:

1. will not be used in invasive procedures;

2. will not be inserted into body orifices nor be used in a sterile procedure

Surgical Asepsis

All microbial life, pathogens and nonpathogens, are destroyed before an invasive procedure is performed. Surgical asepsis and sterile technique are often used interchangeably.

Four methods of sterilization

1. Gas sterilization: often used for wheelchairs and hospital beds. Useful in hospitals, but costly for the office.

2. Dry heat sterilization: requires higher temperature that steam sterilization but longer exposure times. Used for instruments that easily corrodes.

3. Chemical sterilization - uses the same chemical used for chemical disinfection, but the exposure time is longer.

4. Steam sterilization (autoclave) - uses steam under pressure to obtain high temperature of 250-254F with exposure times of 20-40 minutes depending on the item being sterilized.

Handwashing

Hand washing is the most important means of preventing the spread of infection. A routine hand wash procedure uses plain soap to remove soil and transient bacteria. Hand antisepsis requires

the use of antimicrobial soap to remove, kill or inhibit transient microorganisms. It is important that all healthcare personnel learn proper hand washing procedures.

Barrier Protection

Protective clothing provides a barrier against infection. Used properly, it will provide protection to the person wearing it; disposed of properly it will assist in the spread of infection. Learning how to put on and remove protective clothing is vital to insure the health and wellness of the person wearing the PPE. PPE's or personal protective equipment includes:

Masks

Goggles

Face Shields

Respirator

Isolation Precautions

For many years, the CDC recommended universal precautions, which is a method of infection control that assumed that all human blood and body fluids were potentially infectious. The CDC issued a revised guidelines consisting of two tiers or levels of precautions: Standard Precautions and Transmission-Based Precautions.

Standard Precautions

This is an infection control method designed to prevent direct contact with blood and other body fluids and tissues by using barrier protection and work control practices.

Under the standard precautions, all patients are presumed to be infective for blood-borne pathogens. Infection control practices to be used with all patients. These replace universal precautions and body substance isolation. They are used when there is a possibility of contact with any of the following:

- Blood

- All body fluids, secretions, and excretions (except sweat), regardless of whether or not they contain visible blood

- Nonintact skin

- Mucous membranes designed to reduce the risk of transmission of microorganisms from both

- Recognized and unrecognized sources of infections.

The standard precautions are:

Wear gloves when collecting and handling blood, body fluids, or tissue specimen.

Wear face shields when there is a danger for splashing on mucous membranes.

Dispose of all needles and sharp objects in puncture-proof containers without recapping.

Transmission- Based Precautions the second tier of precautions and are to be used when the patient is known or suspected of being infected with contagious disease. They are to be used in addition to standard precautions. All types of isolation are condensed into three categories:

Contact precautions: are designed to reduce the risk of transmission of microorganisms by direct or indirect contact. Direct-contact transmission involves skin-to-skin contact and physical transfer of microorganisms to a susceptible host from an infected or colonized person. Indirect-contact

transmission involves contact with a contaminated intermediate object in the patient's environment.

Airborne precautions: are designed to reduce the risk of airborne transmission of infectious agents. Microorganisms carried in this manner can be dispersed widely by air currents and may become inhaled by or deposited on a susceptible host within the same room or over a longer distance from the source patient. Special air handling and ventilation are required to prevent airborne transmission.

Contact precautions: are designed to reduce the risk of transmission of microorganisms by direct or indirect contact. Direct-contact transmission involves skin-to-skin contact and physical transfer of microorganisms to a susceptible host from an infected or colonized person. Indirect-contact

transmission involves contact with a contaminated intermediate object in the patient's environment.

Airborne precautions: are designed to reduce the risk of airborne transmission of infectious agents. Microorganisms carried in this manner can be dispersed widely by air currents and may become inhaled by or deposited on a susceptible host within the same room or over a longer distance from the source patient. Special air handling and ventilation are required to prevent airborne transmission.

Section One Questions
1. Which of the following is an example of the duties of a nurse assistant?
   a. Handling basic paperwork
   b. Taking the vital signs of the patients
   c. Assisting in bed bath
   d. All of the above are functions of a CNA

2. What is a thermometer used for?
   a. Assessing the pulse of a patient
   b. Measuring blood pressure of a patient
   c. Measuring body temperature
   d. Assessing the responsiveness of a patient

3. An oral thermometer produces a reading of 101 degrees Fahrenheit. This patient is:
   a. Febrile
   b. Afebrile
   c. Normal
   d. None of the above

4. A fever that remains constant is:
   a. Remittent
   b. Afebrile
   c. Continuous
   d. Intermittent

5. Who should have their temperatures taken orally?
   a. Elderly patients
   b. Patients receiving oxygen
   c. Teenage patients
   d. Patients with broken ribs

6. Which patients should not have temperatures taken rectally?
   a. Patients with NG tubes
   b. Patients with diarrhea
   c. Infants
   d. Patients who smoke

7. How should a pulse be taken?
   a. With the first two or three fingers for about thirty seconds
   b. With the third and fourth finger on the femoral artery
   c. With the thumb on the jugular

d. With the thumb on the brachial artery

8. Which of the following counts as a respiration?
   a. An inhale
   b. An inhale and an exhale
   c. An exhale
   d. A cough

9. The apical pulse is taken:
   a. With the first and second finger
   b. Over the apex of the heart with the palm of the hand
   c. Over the apex of the heart with a stethoscope
   d. None of the above

10. The apical pulse is especially useful in:
    a. Infants or small children
    b. In the elderly
    c. In patients with brittle bones
    d. In patients going into fibrillation

11. When taking a pulse you should feel:
    a. On the radial artery which is located on the same side as the patient's pinky
    b. On the brachial artery on the back side of the arm
    c. On the temporal artery located on the forehead
    d. On the radial artery located on the same side as the patient's thumb

12. Tachypnea is characterized by:
    a. A rate of breathing greater than 40 breaths per minute
    b. A rate of breathing less than 10 breaths per minute
    c. A rate of breathing greater than 100 breaths per minute
    d. A rate of breathing less than 5 breaths per minute

13. A patient has a fever that has been fluctuating all day. However, the fever never returns to a baseline or a normal temperature. This is considered:
    a. Continuous fever
    b. Intermittent fever
    c. Remittent fever
    d. Afebrile fever

14. Apnea occurs when:
    a. The patient permanently stops breathing
    b. The patient temporarily has complete absence of breath
    c. The patient is in hysteria
    d. The patient is breathing normally

15. Bradypnea:
    a. Occurs when a patient hyperventilates
    b. Has a breathing rate of greater than 40 breaths per minute
    c. Is normal during a sleeping state
    d. Is never normal

16. Depth of respiration refers to:
    a. Number of breaths per minutes
    b. Amount of air inspired and expired
    c. Number of heartbeats per minute
    d. Amount of blood pumped through the heart per minute

17. Hypoventilation refers to a time when:
    a. Reduced air enters the lungs
    b. Increased air enters the lungs
    c. Normal amounts of air enters the lungs
    d. No air enters the lungs

18. Hypoventilation results in:
    a. Excess oxygen in the blood and decreased carbon dioxide in the blood
    b. Excess nitrogen in the blood and decreased carbon dioxide
    c. Decreased nitrogen in the blood and increased oxygen in the blood
    d. Decreased oxygen in the blood and increased carbon dioxide

19. Blood pressure can be described as:
    a. The distance pressurized blood will travel
    b. The amount of stress that veins can safely handle
    c. The amount of force exerted by blood on peripheral arteries
    d. None of the above

20. An instrument that measures blood pressure is known as a:
    a. Hypometer
    b. Sphygmomanometer
    c. Barometer
    d. Mercometer

21. Which artery does the blood pressure cuff center over?
    a. Jugular artery
    b. Femoral artery
    c. Antecubital artery
    d. Brachial artery

22. Failure to properly place the cuff can lead to:
    a. False diagnosis of high or low blood pressure
    b. Rupture of the veins

c. Accurate diagnosis of high or low blood pressure

d. Discomfort

23. Cuffs that are too small or narrow can lead to:
    a. Unusually low blood pressure readings
    b. Abnormal heart rate readings
    c. Unusually high blood pressure readings
    d. All of the above

24. Anthropometric measurements refers to:
    a. Measurements of the heart and lungs
    b. Comparative measurements of the body
    c. Comparative measurements of lung function
    d. All of the above

25. During the examination, the medical assistant will be responsible for:
    a. Room and patient preparation
    b. Patient examination
    c. Patient treatment
    d. Room maintenance

26. Which of the following does the physician use to make a diagnosis?
    a. Patient history
    b. Lab tests
    c. Physical examination
    d. All of the above

27. How would someone examine a patient using palpation?
    a. Listening to breath sounds
    b. Tapping on a patient's chest to listen to the sounds
    c. Feeling a pulse
    d. All of the above

28. Which position is the most commonly used for patient examination?
    a. The vertical recumbent position
    b. The horizontal flat dorsal position
    c. Vertical pineal dorsal position
    d. The horizontal recumbent position

29. Which of the following is used for pelvic exams?
    a. Dorsal lithotomy position
    b. The horizontal recumbent position
    c. The vertical recumbent position
    d. Dilliad's position

30. A patient comes in for an exam. The patient is having trouble breathing. Which position do you place the patient in?
    a. Vertical recumbent position
    b. Fowler's position
    c. Dilliard's position
    d. Any of the above

31. Which position is used for a rectal exam?
    a. Fowler's position
    b. Prone position
    c. Sim's position
    d. Dilliard's position

32. Most accidents occur because:
    a. The patient does not cooperate
    b. Rules are overlooked or ignored
    c. Healthcare professionals don't care
    d. None of the above

33. Which of the following is an example of a hazard in the healthcare setting?
    a. Electrical hazards
    b. Biological hazards
    c. Chemical hazards
    d. All of the above

34. A coworker has noticed a stripped cord connected to a bed. This is an example of:
    a. Electrical hazards
    b. Biological hazards
    c. Chemical hazards
    d. Neurological hazards

35. Someone has left out some strong cleaning supplies. This is an example of:
    a. Electrical hazards
    b. Biological hazards
    c. Chemical hazards
    d. Neurological hazards

36. Someone has left out an uncapped, used sharp. This is an example of:
    a. Electrical hazards
    b. Biological hazards
    c. Chemical hazards
    d. Neurological hazards

37. A coworker has cut himself badly on a jagged piece of metal. You should:
    a. Have the coworker lie down
    b. Pour disinfectant on the wound
    c. Apply pressure and elevate the wound
    d. Perform CPR

38. A patient is on the floor with cold/clammy skin, blank expression, and shallow breathing. This patient possibly is suffering from:
    a. Shock
    b. Stroke
    c. Heart attack
    d. Sun poisoning

39. CPR stands for:
    a. Cardio-Palpitative Resuscitation
    b. Carotid-Pulmonary Recognizance
    c. Cardio-Pulmonary Resuscitation
    d. Carotid-Palliative Recognizance

40. An influenza virus is an example of:
    a. An agent
    b. A portal of exit
    c. A mode of transmission
    d. A portal of entry

41. Which of the following is not an example of a portal of entry?
    a. A scratch on the hand
    b. Intact skin
    c. A mucous membrane
    d. Respiratory tract

42. Which of the following is not an example of a mode of transmission?
    a. Wearing gloves
    b. Being sneezed on
    c. Contact with blood
    d. Touching an infected surface

43. Which of the following means "the destruction of pathogenic microorganisms after they leave the body"?
    a. Vector transmission
    b. Asymmetry
    c. Medical Asepsis
    d. Organ Sepsis

44. When disinfecting items you should:
    a. Use chemicals on every item to be disinfected
    b. Put everything into a cleaning oven
    c. Wipe everything down with water
    d. Use chemicals only on inanimate objects

45. Which item would not be eligible to be cleaned with boiling water?
    a. An oral thermometer
    b. A pair of utility scissors
    c. A reflex hammer
    d. A mug

46. Surgical instruments are placed in an autoclave. This is an example of:
    a. Dry heat sterilization
    b. Chemical sterilization
    c. Steam sterilization
    d. Gas sterilization

47. A wheelchair is placed in a chamber for sterilization. This is most likely an example of:
    a. Dry heat sterilization
    b. Chemical sterilization
    c. Steam sterilization
    d. Gas sterilization

48. The most important way of fighting infection is:
    a. Dry heat sterilization
    b. Hand washing
    c. Cleaning things with bleach
    d. All of the above

49. You must wear a face shield for performing a procedure. This is an example of:
    a. Isolation
    b. Medical asepsis
    c. Barrier protection
    d. Contact asepsis

50. Standard precautions include which of the following?
    a. Wearing gloves
    b. Wearing face shields when necessary
    c. Disposing of sharps without recapping
    d. All of the above

51. In order to prevent airborne diseases from spreading you should use:
    a. Universal precautions

b. Contact precautions
c. Airborne precautions
d. All of the above

52. You catch a cold after you drink after your daughter. This is an example of:
   a. Airborne contamination
   b. Indirect contact transmission
   c. Direct contact transmission
   d. Vector transmission

53. A patient contracted a disease from the hospital. This is an example of:
   a. A nosocomial infection
   b. Direct contact transmission
   c. Barrier protection
   d. A susceptible host

54. A child develops a rash after playing closely with another child. This could be an example of:
   a. Direct contact transmission
   b. Airborne transmission
   c. Vector transmission
   d. Indirect contact transmission

55. A virus is an example of a:
   a. Susceptible host
   b. An agent
   c. A vector
   d. Portal of exit

56. Standard precautions are aimed at:
   a. Preventing the spread of infectious agents as they exit the reservoir
   b. Preventing the spread of infectious as they enter the susceptible host
   c. Preventing the spread of infectious agents as they travel through the air
   d. None of the above

57. When a person appears to be in shock you should:
   a. Have the person sit up and elevate the arms
   b. Have the person stand up and elevate the arms
   c. Have the person lay down and elevate the feet
   d. None of the above

58. When should you wash your hands?
   a. Before and after speaking with the patient
   b. Before and after entering a room
   c. After eating and using the bathroom

d. After leaving the hospital

59. To avoid chemical hazards you should always:
    a. Store chemicals with non-hazardous materials
    b. Pour chemicals into clear bottles
    c. Label all chemicals with the MSDS
    d. All of the above

60. In order to avoid biological hazards you should:
    a. Incinerate any non-cleanable materials
    b. Sterilize any materials that can be sterilized
    c. Wash hands before and after each procedure
    d. All of the above

61. To avoid electrical hazards you should:
    a. Never use extension cords
    b. Replace any cords that are bare or have the wire showing
    c. Unplug electrical equipment before servicing
    d. All of the above

62. When an accident occurs you should:
    a. Attempt to clean up the mess before anyone notices
    b. Talk about it with a co-worker
    c. Report it to a supervisor
    d. Leave it for someone else

63. A patient needs to be examined in the posterior aspect. Which position should you use for this patient?
    a. Trendelenburg
    b. Prone position
    c. Sim's position
    d. None of the above

64. Which of the following would a medical assistant do for the patient?
    a. Collect vitals
    b. Explain the procedure
    c. Positioning and draping the patient
    d. All of the above

65. Which of the following is not an anthropometric measurement?
    a. Lucidity
    b. Weight
    c. Height
    d. Head circumference

66. How fast should a blood pressure cuff deflate?
    a. 1-2 mmHg per second
    b. 2-3 mmHg per second
    c. 4-5 mmHg per second
    d. 6-7 mmHg per second

67. A state where increased air is entering the lungs is called:
    a. Hypopnea
    b. Hyperpnoea
    c. Hyperventilation
    d. Hypoventilation

68. Cheyne-Stokes refers to:
    a. Regular pattern of irregular breathing
    b. Irregular pattern of regular breathing
    c. Regular pattern of regular breathing
    d. Irregular pattern of irregular breathing

69. Orthopnea refers to:
    a. Trouble breathing because of problems with the rib bones
    b. Regular breathing in an inverted position
    c. Difficulty breathing when not upright
    d. Difficulty breathing when upright

70. Apnea refers to:
    a. A period of increased breathing, then returning to normal
    b. A period if no breath
    c. A period if decreased breath depth
    d. None of the above

71. When using a rectal thermometer:
    a. All patients are eligible for rectal thermometers
    b. Only babies should have rectal temperatures taken
    c. Only elderly patients should have rectal temperatures taken
    d. Patients with heart disease should not have rectal temperatures taken

72. If a patient has just been drinking or smoking you should:
    a. Take temperature orally anyway
    b. Wait thirty minutes and then take his/her temperature
    c. Wait ten minutes and then take temperature rectally
    d. None of the above

73. A patient is described as afebrile. This patient is:
    a. Having heart trouble
    b. Having breathing trouble

c. Has a normal body temperature

d. Has fertility problems

74. A patient has an axillary temperature of 98 degrees Fahrenheit. This patient:
    a. Has a normal body temperature
    b. Has a low body temperature
    c. Has a high body temperature
    d. Should be tested with an oral thermometer

75. Which of the following is not a place to take a temperature?
    a. Axillary area
    b. Rectal area
    c. Antecubital area
    d. Ear

76. Social history includes:
    a. Summary of family health problems
    b. Lifestyle
    c. Past surgeries
    d. Chief complaint

77. Medical history includes:
    a. Past surgeries
    b. Major illnesses
    c. Medications
    d. All of the above

78. Family history includes:
    a. Health problems of parents
    b. Past surgeries
    c. Lifestyle
    d. Major illnesses

79. A systematic check of each organ and system along with documenting positive
    and negative results is called a:
    a. Review of the body
    b. Review of systems
    c. Review of the patient
    d. None of the above

80. A Medical Assistant might:
    a. Collect specimens
    b. Instruct a patient about medications
    c. Gather vitals

d. All of the above

81. Medical assistants do not:
    a. Make a diagnosis
    b. Assist the physician
    c. Dispose of contaminated supplies
    d. Prepare patients for XRays

82. Medical assistants might:
    a. Do medical transcription
    b. Maintain medical records
    c. Manage finances
    d. All of the above

83. An explanation of the chief complaint along with the symptoms and duration is part of:
    a. Social history
    b. Family history
    c. History of present illness
    d. Medical history

84. Which of the following is not a vital sign?
    a. Respiration
    b. Weight
    c. Pulse
    d. Temperature

85. Which of the following is the least accurate way to attain a temperature?
    a. Rectally
    b. Orally
    c. Ear
    d. Axillary

86. The normal pulse ranges between:
    a. 20 and 40 BPM
    b. 30 and 70 BPM
    c. 60 and 100 BPM
    d. 90 and 130 BPM

87. When taking a blood pressure with a stethoscope and a sphygmomanometer:
    a. Note the level at which two consecutive beats occur and the level at which all sounds disappear
    b. Note the level at which the blood pressure cuff becomes too tight
    c. Note the level at which the cuff completely deflates

d. None of the above

88. To avoid biological hazards you should:
    a. Always wear gloves
    b. Disinfect the work area
    c. Wash hands
    d. All of the above

89. A person sneezes and germs are spread through drops across the room. This is an example of:
    a. Airborne transmission
    b. Droplet transmission
    c. Contact transmission
    d. All of the above

90. A person is blankly staring, has a rapid and weak pulse, and increased, shallow breathing. This person may be suffering from:
    a. Cheyne-Stokes
    b. Shock
    c. Stroke
    d. Hematoma

91. If it is necessary to use a bleach solution for disinfecting it should be diluted:
    a. 1 bleach : 1 water
    b. 2 bleach : 1 water
    c. 4 bleach : 1 water
    d. 1 bleach : 10 water

92. Airborne precautions are used to isolate:
    a. All patients that might have any contagion
    b. Any patients that might pose a direct contact threat
    c. Any patient that might offer airborne infection
    d. Only young and elderly patients

93. Contact precautions are used when:
    a. The patient might have a disease that is spread through direct contact
    b. A patient might have an airborne disease
    c. A patient might have a droplet disease
    d. None of the above

94. Standard precautions are:
    a. Precautions used only for contagious patients
    b. Precautions used only when the caregiver is ill
    c. Precautions used on all patients

d. Precautions used only on foreign patients

95. Which of the following is the most important and most basic way of preventing disease transmission?
    a. Face masks
    b. Gloves
    c. Face shields
    d. Hand washing

96. Dry heat sterilization would be used for:
    a. Cleaning hands
    b. Cleaning wheelchairs
    c. Cleaning instruments that easily corrode
    d. Cleaning beds

97. A fungi is an example of a:
    a. Vector
    b. Agent
    c. Reservoir
    d. Host

98. A person is bleeding. This is an example of:
    a. Susceptible host
    b. Shock
    c. External hemorrhaging
    d. All of the above

99. When should you wash your hands?
    a. Before and after speaking with the patient
    b. Before and after entering a room
    c. After eating and using the bathroom
    d. After leaving the hospital

100.   Which of the following pressurizes steam in order to sterilize?
    a. Chemical sterilization
    b. Dry heat sterilization
    c. Steam sterilization
    d. Water sterilization

Section One Answers

1. D
2. C
3. A
4. C
5. B
6. B
7. A
8. B
9. C
10. A
11. D
12. A
13. C
14. B
15. C
16. B
17. A
18. D
19. C
20. B
21. D
22. A
23. C
24. B
25. A
26. D
27. B
28. D
29. A
30. B
31. C
32. B
33. D
34. A
35. C
36. B
37. C
38. A
39. C
40. A
41. B

42. A
43. C
44. D
45. A
46. C
47. D
48. B
49. C
50. D
51. C
52. B
53. A
54. A
55. B
56. A
57. C
58. B
59. C
60. D
61. D
62. C
63. B
64. D
65. A
66. B
67. C
68. A
69. C
70. B
71. D
72. B
73. C
74. A
75. C
76. B
77. D
78. A
79. B
80. D
81. A
82. D
83. C
84. B
85. D
86. C

87. A
88. D
89. B
90. B
91. D
92. C
93. A
94. C
95. D
96. C
97. B
98. C
99. B
100.   C

Patient Care Procedures

Care of the surgical patient

A. Perform tasks from pre-operative checklist

  1. Showering, bathing

  2. Enemas - per hospital policy

  3. Nonsterile douche - per hospital policy

  4. Shave prep

  5. Hospital gown

  6. NPO after midnight or as ordered by physician

  7. Vital signs

  8. Remove dentures, if ordered.

  9. Remove prostheses (i.e., hearing aids, glasses, contact lenses, splints, braces, artificial parts).

  10. Remove jewelry, hair pins, makeup.

  11. Tape wedding rings, if allowed.

  12. Assure security of any items of value (i.e., give jewelry to family member with patient's permission).

  13. Have patient empty bladder. Drain Foley if present. Record output.

  14. Notify medication nurse when patient is ready.

  15. Provide for safe environment after pre-operative

medication (i.e., side rails up, safety belt fastened

on gurney, call light in reach).

B. Identify nurse assistant's role in pre-operational checklist

C. Document on the preoperative checklist

Nurse assistant's responsibilities while the patient is in surgery.

A. Prepare the room:

1. Surgical bed

2. Emesis basin

3. Facial tissue

4. Vital sign equipment

5. IV pole

6. Incontinent pads.

B. Collect additional equipment as ordered

1. O_2 equipment

2. Pulse Oximeter

3. Suction

Patient care measures provided in the post-operative phase.

A. Post-operative checks

1. Note time of return.

2. Note level of consciousness.

3. Check dressings for location and condition (dryness).

4. Observe incisions, report any drainage, redness or swelling (assessing and

changing the dressing is the responsibility of the licensed nurse).

5. Check IV for location and observe site for redness, swelling, warmth or drainage.

6. Observe to see that IV is dripping and tubing not kinked.

B. Post-operative care measures

1. Assist in transfer from gurney to bed.

2. Vital signs

   a. Be aware of changes in vital signs that signal hemorrhage, i.e., decreasing blood pressure and increasing pulse.

   b. Elevated temperature may signal infection.

   c. Report abnormalities to licensed personnel promptly.

   d. Pulse oximetry

3. Observations

   a. Comfort: degree of pain or other discomfort

   b. Safety: side rails, call light within reach

   c. Equipment: report if disconnected or malfunctioning

   d. Changes in behavior: confusion, disorientation, agitation

   e. Changes in skin color: pallor, gray, blue-tinged

   f. Nausea, vomiting

   g. Bowel activity, passing gas

C. Care measures to prevent complications

1. Encourage

   a. Turn, cough and deep breathing

   b. Incentive spirometer

   c. Leg exercises

2. Apply TED hose and sequential compression de-vices, if ordered.

3. Reposition at least every 2 hours to prevent hypo-static pneumonia.

4. Apply binders, if ordered.

5. Assist with dangling and initial ambulation, as ordered

6. Review Hazards of Immobility and Role of the Nurse Assistant.

D. **Complications of Immobility: Deep Vein Thrombosis (DVT)** – blood clot in lower extremity

   1. General Information

      a. Deep vein thrombus (DVT) or blood clot occurs in pelvic veins or in deep veins of the lower extremities in post-operative patients. The incidence of DVT varies between 10% and 40% depending upon how serious the surgery is and how many other medical problems the patient has.

      b. DVT is most common following hip surgery, then prostate surgery and general thoracic or abdominal surgery.

      c. Blood clots located above the knee are considered the major source of pulmonary emboli (a blood clot that dislodges from the vein wall and travels to the lungs, causing death of lung tissue)

   2. Causes

      a. Pooling of blood in lower extremities (venous stasis)

      b. Inactivity and immobility

      c. Some medical conditions (stroke, heart attack, congestive heart failure)

      d. Obesity

      e. Varicose veins

      f. Surgery and anesthesia

      g. Age, particularly over 65 years

    h. Damage to or stretching of blood vessels during surgery or trauma

    i. Central venous catheters, pacemaker wires

    j. Previous DVT

    k. Increased tendency of blood to clot (some diseases like cancer, blood diseases, protein deficiency in malnourishment, dehydration)

    l. Oral contraceptives and estrogen replacement

    m. Smoking

3. Symptoms of DVT

    a. Often have no symptoms

    b. Pain or cramp in the calf or thigh, progressing to painful swelling of entire leg

    c. Slight fever, chills, perspiration (diaphoresis), generalized feeling of discomfort

    d. Painful tenderness over inner thigh

4. Prevention

    a. Increased activity, early ambulation after surgery, frequent and proper repositioning

    b. Range of motion

    c. Anti-embolic stockings (TED hose)

    d. Purpose of anti-embolic stockings

        1) To help prevent formation of blood clots

        2) To promote increased blood flow in the legs by compression of deep veins

        3) To improve venous return from the legs to the heart maintenance of anti-embolic stockings

4) Properly sized stockings need to be removed daily during bathing to inspect condition of skin. Do not leave off more than 30 minutes.

5) Wash stockings every 2 to 3 days to remove bodily secretions.

6) For patient's information at home, the stockings can usually be machine washed on delicate and machine dried on low for 15 to 20 minutes.

7) With correct care stockings last 3 to 4 months.

8) Do not use ointments on the leg when using anti-embolic stockings.

e. Sequential compressions sleeves or devices

f. Adequate fluids

g. Avoid dependent positioning of lower extremities (elevate legs when up in chair, avoid knee gatch when in bed).

h. Doctor may order anticoagulants for licensed nurse to administer; observe for signs of bleeding or bruising.

i. Observe for pain in calf, fever or chills, painful swelling of leg, tenderness over inner thigh.

j. Report any shortness of breath or chest pain immediately to the licensed nurse.

E. *Nursing Alert*

1. *A complaint of slight soreness of the calf is never ignored. Blood clots in the calf or thigh can break loose and travel to the lungs (pulmonary embolism). This is life threatening.*

2. *Close observation of patients and attention to their complaints of pain or discomfort is very important.*

3. *Report this to the licensed nurse.*

4. Never rub or massage the lower legs.

SEQUENTIAL COMPRESSION DEVICES

Several types of devices are available that supply intermittent compression over the lower leg, thigh or foot. Each device aids in the return of venous blood and helps prevent deep vein thrombosis and pulmonary embolism. They are usually used in addition to anti-embolic stockings.

The typical type of sequential compression device consists of a vinyl or plastic sleeve that fits over the foot, lower leg or thigh. It may come as a tube or as a wrap style that fastens with Velcro. It is attached to a control unit that is placed on the floor under the bed. The control unit has a small pump that inflates and deflates channels in the sleeve to provide increasing and decreasing pressure. Connecting tubing attaches to the sleeve and to the control unit completing a closed system. The pressure can be adjusted according to facility policy or as ordered by the physician.

The device should be removed at least twice daily for 20 to 30 minutes to allow for ambulation, bathing and inspection of the skin. Sequential compression devices are usually worn at least 3 days after surgery or until the patient is up and ambulating regularly or as long as the doctor orders.

EQUIPMENT:

1. Sequential compression sleeves

2. Connectors

3. Control unit

CRITERIA:

Safely cares for the patient on a sequential compression device

1. Wash hands, identify patient, introduce self, explain procedure and provide for privacy.

2. Position patient, exposing one leg at a time for application of sequential sleeve.

3. Align leg on the open sleeve according to instructions included in package.

4. Wrap the sleeve securely around the patient's leg and fasten the Velcro tabs, thigh section first. Make sure that no wrinkles are in the plastic of the sleeve and that at least two fingers can be inserted between the patient's leg and the sleeve.

5. Make sure the control unit is turned off.

6. Attach the connector on the sleeve to the correct end of the connector tubing. Check carefully to be certain there are no kinks or twists in the tubing.

7. Attach the other end of the connector tubing to the control unit.

8. Turn the power on and adjust or monitor the pressure according to your facility's policy.

9. Remain with the patient for at least a complete cycle to monitor comfort and the functioning of the unit.

10. Sleeves should be removed if the patient experiences numbness, tingling or leg pain. Notify licensed nurse if any of these symptoms occur.

11. Document time of application, type of device, condition of skin and comfort of patient.

PRECAUTIONS:

1. Do not apply to any patient experiencing skin rash or poor circulation evidenced by bluish-red coloring of lower legs and feet, sores on lower legs or feet, severe edema or leg pain, edema of the lungs from congestive heart failure.
2. Make sure that connectors and sleeves are properly applied.
3. Monitor the patient's condition frequently, according to facility policy.

SINGLE LEG APPLICATION:

1. Most brands of sequential compression devices can be used on only one leg, if necessary.
2. The unused sleeve is kept in the plastic wrapper and attached to the second sleeve connector.
3. The compression action of the pump will not work unless there is a closed system. By keeping the unused sleeve folded in the wrapper, the system will be able to reach the proper compression.

MEASURING AND APPLICATION OF ANTI-EMBOLIC STOCKINGS

EQUIPMENT:

1. Tape measure (new one for each patient)

2. Scratch pad, order form or requisition form from Central Supply

3. Anti-embolic stockings (TED stockings or other brands)

CRITERIA:

Correctly measures and applies anti-embolic stockings

A. Thigh length

1. Measure upper thigh circumference at gluteal furrow.

2. Measure calf circumference at widest area.

3. Measure length from gluteal furrow to base of heel.

4. Consult sizing chart from Central Supply or TED stockings order pad, if available.

    ○ TED thigh length with belt stocking fit a thigh circumference of up to 32 inches.

    ○ TED thigh length stocking fit a maximum thigh circumference of 25 inches.

B. Knee length

1. Measure calf circumference at widest area.

2. Measure length from bend of knee to base of heel.

C. Medicare usually covers two pair to insure that compression goes uninterrupted during laundering care. Check with the RN to see if one or two pair should be ordered.

D. Different brands of anti-embolic elastic stockings are available. Each pair will have a large round hole in the toe to check for circulation. In some brands the hole will be on top of the toes and some will have the hole open under the toes.

APPLICATION OF ANTI-EMBOLIC STOCKINGS:

1. Obtain correct size of anti-embolic stockings.

2. Wash hands, identify patient, introduce self, explain procedure and provide for privacy.

3. With patient lying down, expose one leg at a time for application of stocking.

4. Insert hand into stocking as far as the heel pocket.

5. Grasp center of heel pocket and turn stocking inside out to heel area.

6. Position stocking over foot and heel. Be sure patient's heel is centered in heel pocket.

7. Pull a few inches of the stocking up around the ankle and calf.

8. Continue pulling the stocking up the leg. If there is a change in the sheerness of the stocking material, it should fall between 1" to 2" below the bend of the knee.

9. As thigh portion of the stocking is applied, start rotating stocking inward so gusset is centered over femoral artery. Gusset is placed slightly towards the inside of the leg. When using thigh length stockings, the top band rests in the gluteal furrow.

10. Smooth out wrinkles.

11. Align inspection toe to fall at base of toes either on the top or underneath, depending on brand.

12. Instruct patient on proper positioning of stockings to insure that he/she will not reposition the stockings incorrectly.

13. Repeat procedure on opposite leg.

14. Wash hands.

15. Report procedure and document size and style of stocking applied.

16. Document when stockings are removed along with condition of skin.

17. Report any tenderness in calves, thighs or toes.

TURNING A SURGICAL PATIENT

EQUIPMENT:

1. Pillows

2. Lift sheet

CRITERIA:

Safely turns a surgical patient

Instruct patient in splinting incision for comfort.

1. Obtain patient activity orders from licensed nurse.

2. Instruct patient in splinting incision for comfort.

3. Make sure that bed wheels are locked, curtains are pulled around bed for privacy and bed is raised to highest level for good body mechanics.

4. Lower head of bed if patient's condition allows.

5. Using good body mechanics, turn patient.

6. Position patient for comfort and in good body alignment.

   a. Place pillow under head.

   b. Position a pillow against back for support.

c. Place a pillow in front of the bottom leg and place the top leg on top of the

   pillow

   in a flexed position.

d. Check lower shoulder to make sure it is not squeezed in an abnormal position.

   Reach under shoulder and pull forward gently until patient is comfortable.

e. Support upper arm and hand with a pillow for comfort, either in front of the

   patient or back on the pillow behind the patient.

f. If abdominal incision is pulling, may place pillow under side of abdomen.

7. Place the signal cord within reach; raise side rails, lower bed to lowest position, open

   curtains around bed.

DANGLE AND AMBULATE A SURGICAL PATIENT

CRITERIA:

Safely dangles and ambulates a surgical patient

1. Check patient's pulse, blood pressure and respirations.

2. Assist patient to side of bed and put on non-slip slippers.

3. Assist patient to pivot and sit at side of bed.

4. Support patient and observe for abnormal signs.

5. Assist patient to put on robe.

6. Apply gait belt if allowed.

7. Assist the patient to stand.

8. Stand at patient's side until steady, holding the gait belt in the middle of the

   patient's back.

9. Stand slightly behind patient, on weak side, if applicable.

10. Encourage patient to walk with head up, standing erect.

11. Observe for signs of activity intolerance (increased pain, shortness of breath, pallor, diaphoresis).

12. Return patient to bed and make sure patient is safe and comfortable.

13. Report distance patient walked and how well patient tolerated activity to licensed nurse.

14. If patient has an IV, may need two people to assist with ambulation.

HAZARDS OF IMMOBILITY AND ROLE OF THE NURSE ASSISTANT

1. Cardiovascular complications - blood clots, orthostatic hypotension, increased work on the heart

- Remind patient to do exercises given by the physical and occupational therapist.

  - Encourage intake of adequate fluids to prevent dehydration.

  - Early ambulation as allowed.

  - Proper positioning and avoidance of pressure on blood vessels.

  - Do not massage the calf of the leg.

2. Respiratory complications – slow and shallow respirations, pooling of respiratory secretions, hypostatic pneumonia, pulmonary embolism

  - Remind patient to turn, cough, take deep breaths and to use incentive spirometer.

  - Increase activity as soon as allowed by patient's condition and doctor's orders.

  - Encourage fluids as allowed to keep lung secretions thinned.

3. Gastrointestinal complications – poor appetite, poor nutrition, constipation, fecal impaction

- Offer adequate fluids.

  - Prevent incontinence by timely offering of the bedpan and early mobility for access to the bathroom.

  - Monitor patient's appetite and ask RN to assess need for a dietician consult.

4. Urinary system complications – urinary retention, incontinence, increased risk of kidney stones, urinary tract infections

- Keep accurate record of intake and output.

- Observe for pain in the back and blood in the urine.

- Observe for signs of urinary tract infection: pain with urination, frequent urination of small amounts, feeling the need to urinate all the time, concentrated or cloudy urine.

5. Musculoskeletal system complications – muscle wasting and atrophy, stiff joints, decreased balance, loss of endurance, osteoporosis, contractures, foot drop

- Perform passive ROM exercises for patients who are unable to do them, and instruct patients who are able to do active or active-assistive ROM.

- Position patients properly in bed, using good body alignment.

- Remind and reinforce any exercises given to patient by physical or occupational therapists and RN.

6. Integumentary system complications – pressure on bony prominences, impaired circulation to skin layers, skin breakdown, pressure ulcers, infections

- Observe for any sign of redness or sores on the skin.

- Keep skin clean and dry.

- Keep bedding free of wrinkles and crumbs.

- Turn patient at least every 2 hours to reduce pressure on bony prominence

Gastro-intestinal care

Common diseases/disorders of the GI system.

A. Congenital: cleft palate

B. Inflammation: stomatitis, esophagitis, gastro-enteritis, colitis, cholecystitis, pancreatitis, hepatitis, cholelithiasis

C. Ulceration: stomach, duodenum, colon

D. Hernias: inguinal, umbilical, hiatal, inicisional.

E. Tumors: benign, malignant

F. Bowel disorders: distension, diarrhea, constipation, and impaction

Patient preparation for GI diagnostic tests.

A. Radiology Testing

    1. UGI

    2. Small bowel series

    3. Gall bladder series

    4. Barium enema

B. Direct Visualization

    1. Colonoscopy/sigmoidoscopy

    2. Esophagogastroduodenoscopy (EGD)

    3. Gastroscopy

    4. Endoscopy

    5. Swallowing evaluation

    6. Gastric sampling

    7. Ultrasound

C. Preparing the patient for diagnostic tests

   1. NPO for at least eight hours (or as ordered)

   2. Give enemas as ordered.

   3. Laxatives given by licensed nurse as ordered.

Special diets as ordered

A. Purpose of enemas: to aid in illumination during x-rays, before surgery, before deliveries, before direct visualization tests, for bowel retraining, to relieve constipation, to expel flatus, to instill medicine.

B. Types of enemas

   1. Cleansing: SSE, TWE, saline, Fleet's phosphosoda.

   2. Retention: medicinal, nutritional, Fleet's oil retention.

   3. Return Flow: Harris flush (HF).

A. Purpose of the sitz bath.

   1. Cleansing

   2. Heat

Healing after perineal/rectal surgery or infant delivery

A. Abnormal signs and symptoms to report to licensed nurse.

   1. Weakness

   2. Rapid, weak pulse

   3. Low blood pressure

   4. Rapid or labored respirations

5. Fatigue

6. Dizziness

7. Fainting

8. Bleeding (coffee grounds emesis, black, tarry stools, rectal bleeding)

9. Change in drainage

10. Change in stool

The difference in care measures between hemodialysis and peritoneal dialysis.

A. Hemodialysis:

1. Procedure that filters and cleans waste products from the blood. It is performed by specially trained RNs.

2. Never take blood pressure in arm with a fistula or shunt

B. Peritoneal dialysis:

1. Removes extra water, waste, and chemicals from body by perfusing sterile solutions through the peritoneal cavity and using the thin membrane that lines the abdominal organs, (peritoneum) as a filter. The dialyzed solution drains out through an abdominal tube.

2. Reporting abnormal signs and symptoms

   a. Fever, nausea/vomiting

   b. Abdominal pain

   c. Redness around the catheter

   d. Change in vital signs

3. Special considerations - no ointments or powder around peritoneal catheter.

4. Prevention of infection

5. Standard precautions

The common sexually transmitted diseases (STDs).

A. Syphilis

B. Gonorrhea

C. Herpes simplex

D. Venereal warts

E. AIDS

F. Chlamydia

    1. Method of transmission:

        a. Mucous membrane to mucous membrane

        b. Mucous membrane to skin

        c. Skin to mucous membrane

    2. Stress nursing considerations: importance of treating all patients with respect and avoiding judgmental attitude regarding patient's lifestyle.

Care measures for the postpartum patient.

A. Observe vaginal discharge for color/odor

    1. Lochia rubra: dark or bright red 3-4 days

    2. Lochia serosa: pinkish brown 10 days

    3. Lochia alba: whitish 2-6 weeks

B. Report number of pads used

C. Observe perineal area for signs of infection

D. Set up sitz bath

E. Assist mom with breastfeeding

F. Watch for signs of urine retention

G. Report bowel activity

H. Burning on urination

I. Leg pain, tenderness, swelling

J. Sadness or feelings of depression

K. Breast pain, tenderness, swelling

Reportable signs and symptoms of postpartum complications.

A. Fever

B. Abdominal or perineal pain

C. Foul smelling vaginal discharge

D. Bleeding from episiotomy or c-section incision

E. Redness/swelling or drainage from c-section incision

F. Saturating sanitary napkin within one hour of application

G. Red lochia after changed to brown

Rules For Body Mechanics

1. Assess the "job" to be done.
2. Use wide base of support – feet – 12 inches apart or shoulder width.
3. Use stronger, larger muscle groups – legs not back and arms.
4. Use correct posture and keep body aligned – back straight, knees bent.
5. Keep objects close to body when lifting or carrying.
6. Never twist your body, turn or pivot feet – face work.
7. Push, slide, or pull heavy objects instead of lifting – pivot.
8. Avoid sudden jerky motions – smooth movements.
9. Use both hands when lifting.

A. Comfort measures for lifting and moving residents.
   1. Inform the resident of what you are doing and why.
   2. Provide privacy.
   3. Raise bed to promote safe body mechanics
   4. Position the resident in proper body alignment.

5.   Use pillows and/or foam pads to support and cushion the resident and protect bony prominences.

6.   Protect all tubing.

7.   Do not slide or drag – skin shearing, abrasion, tear.

B.   Safety measures for lifting and moving residents:

      1.   Assess the task:

            a.   Size up the load.

            b.   Obtain help if needed.

General Review Questions

SECTION ONE

1. _____ are people or organizations paying for health care services

   A. Payers

   B. Providers

   C. Facilities

2. LTC mean

   A. Length of care

   B. Length of cure

   C. Long term care

3. When a person is expected to die from the illness is referred to

   A. Terminal illness

   B. Acute illness

   C. Chronic illness

4. Most conditions seen in long term care facilities are chronic

   A. True

   B. False

5. _____ care is given in hospitals and ambulatory surgical centers.

   A. Acute care

   B. Home healthcare

   C. Adult daycare

6. Which of the following care can be given in a hospital or in a long-term care facility?

   A. Hospice care

   B. Skilled care

   C. Subacute care

7. Preferred provider organizations (PPOs) require that you use a particular doctor or group of doctors except in case of emergency.

   A. True

   B. False

8. Which of the following care is usually for 24 hours?

   A. Skilled care

   B. Outpatient care

9. Daily personal care tasks are called

   A. Active daily living

   B. Activities in daily living

   C. Activities of daily living (ADLs)

10. A thin tube inserted into the body that is used to drain fluids or inject fluid is

    A. Drainage

    B. Catheter

11. Which one of the following is defined as the loss of mental abilities, such as thinking, remembering, reasoning, and communicating?

    A. Dementia

B. Alzheimer's

12. What is a course of action that should be taken every time a certain situation occurs

  A. Procedure

  B. HIPAA

  C. Policy

13. _____ is a method, or way of doing something

  A. Procedure

  B. Policy

  C. Rules

14. Caucasian women make up a high percentage of residents in long term care facilities

  A. True

  B. False

15. Nursing assistance should accept money and gifts from residents

  A. True

  B. False

16. To cite means to

  A. Review a problem though a survey

  B. Find a problem through survey

  C. Create a problem through a survey

17. _____ is an independent not-for-profit organization that evaluates and accredits healthcare organizations.

  A. OSHA

  B. Health Care Finance Administration (HCFA)

  C. Joint Commission on Accreditation of Healthcare Organization(JCAHO)

18. Medicare and Medicaid pay long-term care facilities a fixed amount for services

    A. True

    B. False

19. What is the name of the term given to the process of transforming services for elders so that they are based on the values and practices of the person receiving care.

    A. Culture shock

    B. Culture change

    C. Cultural changes

20. People who live in long term care facilities are usually called

    A. Clients

    B. Residents

C. Patients

SECTION TWO

Match the following

1. CNA _____   A. Direct plan activities for residents to help them socialize and stay physically and mentally active.

2. RN _____   B. Determines residents' needs and helps get them support services such as counseling.

3. LPN/LVN _____   C. Creates diets for resident with specials needs

4. MD/DO _____   D. Help with speech and swallowing problems

5. PT _____   E. Helps residents learn to compensate for disabilities

6. OT _____   F. Evaluates a person and develops a treatment plan to increase movement, improve circulation, promote healing

7. SLP ___   G. Diagnose disease or disability and prescribe treatment

8. RD ___   H. Licensed professional who has completed one to two years of education

9. MSW ___   I. Licensed professional who has completed two to four years of education

10. Activity Director ___   J. Performs delegated tasks such as taking vital signs, provides routine personal care, such as bathing residents and helping with toileting.

11. Professionalism means

    A. How you behave when you are on the job

    B. Having to do with work or a job

    C. Keeping a positive attitude

12. Nursing assistants must be conscientious about documenting observations and procedures

    A. True

    B. False

13. _____ is the ability to understand what is proper and appropriate when dealing with others

    A. Sympathy

    B. Tact

    C. Empathy

Match the following

14. Compassionate ___   A. Put aside your opinions and see each resident as an individual who needs your care

15. Empathy ___   B. Give each resident the same quality care regardless of age, gender, race, ethnicity or condition

16. Sympathy _____   C. Valuing other individuality

17. Conscientious ___   D. Must make and keep commitments

18. Dependable _____   E. Always try to do their best

19. Respectful _____   F. Sharing in the feelings and difficulties of others

20. Unprejudiced _____   G. Entering into feeling of others

21. Tolerant _____   H. Being caring concerned, considerate, empathetic and understanding

22. Which of the following is not included in personal grooming habits

    A. Dressing neatly in a uniform that is washed and ironed

    B. Keep fingernails short, smooth and clean

    C. Wearing little or no makeup

    D. All of the above

23. The chain of command describes the line of authority and helps ensure that the resident receive proper care

    A. True

    B. False

24. _____ defines the things you are allowed to do and how to do them correctly.

    A. Scope of practice

    B. Unprejudiced

    C. Compassionate

    D. Tolerant

Match the following

    25. Diagnosis _____   A. A careful examination to see if the goals are being met

    26. Planning _____   B. Putting the care plan into action

    27. Implementation ___ C. Setting goals and creating a care plan

    28. Evaluation _____   D. Identifying the health problems after looking at all the resident's needs

    29. Plan ahead _____   E. Identifying the most important things to get done

    30. Prioritize _____   F. Best way to help manage your time better

    SECTION THREE

1. The knowledge of right and wrong is

   A. Laws

   B. Rules

   C. Ethics

2. _____ are usually based on ethics

   A. Laws

   B. Rules

   C. Abuse

3. Behaving ethically and following the law and applies to all healthcare providers.

   A. True

   B. False

4. _____ set minimum standards for nursing assistant training

   A. OSHA

   B. OBRA

   C. MDS

5. The _____ is a detailed form with guidelines for assessing residents

   A. OBRA

   B. MDS

   C. OSHA

6. Residents' rights include which of the following

   A. The right to make independent choices

   B. The right to participate in their own care

   C. The right to privacy and confidentiality

D. All of the above

7. _____ is the process by which a person, with the help of a doctor makes informed decisions about his or her healthcare.

A. Living will

B. Informed consent

C. Power of attorney

8. Which of the following is a national non-profit organization founded in 1975 to protect the rights, safety and dignity of long-term care residents

A. Omnibus Budget Reconciliation Act(OBRA)

B. Joint Commission on Accreditation of Healthcare Organization(JCAHO)

C. The National Citizens' Coalition for Nursing Home Reform (NCCNHR)

Match the following

9. Neglect ____ 		A. another tool that help medical providers honor wishes about care

10. Active Neglect ____ 	B. Medical procedures to restart the heart and breathing

11. Passive Neglect __ 	C. A signed dated and witness paper

12. Negligence ____ 	D. Takes effect while the person is still living

13. Malpractice ____ 	E. Legal documents that allow people to choose what medical care they wish to have…

14. Abuse ____ 		F. Any unwelcome sexual advance behavior that creates an offensive working environment

15. Involuntary Seclusion __ 	G. Separating a person from others against the persons will

16. Sexual Harassment ____ 	H. Purposely causing Physical, mental or emotional pain or injury to someone

17. Advanced directives ____ 	I. Occurs when a person is injured due to professional misconduct through negligence

18. Living will ____ 		J. The failure to act to provide the proper care for a resident that result in unintended injury

19. Durable power of attorney ___ K. Unintentionally harming a person physically or by failing to provide care

20. Do-not-resuscitate (DNR) ___ L. Purposely harming a person by failing to provide needed care.

21. Cardiopulmonary resuscitation (CPR) ___ M. Harming a person physically or emotionally by failing to provide needed care

22. _____ are people who are legally required to report suspected or observed abuse or neglect

    A. Mandatory reporters

    B. News reported

    C. Mandated reporters

23. Which of the following is assigned by law as the legal advocate for residents

    A. Protected health information (PHI)

    B. Confidentiality

    C. Ombudsman

24. HIPAA means to

    A. Share private information with family members

    B. Keep private things private

    C. Gives information to the public

25. Only people who give care or process records, should have access to protected health information

    A. True

    B. False

SECTION FOUR

1. _____ is the process of exchanging information with others

A. Compassionate

B. Sympathy

C. Communication

2. The communication process consists of which of the following

   A. Sender, receiver and feedback

   B. Signs, symbols and drawings

   C. Drawings, receiver, sender

3. Verbal communication involves the use of words or sounds, spoken or written

   A. True

   B. False

4. Body language often speaks as words

   A. True

   B. False

5. _____ is the way we communicate without using words

   A. Culture

   B. Nonverbal communication

   C. Verbal communication

6. A _____ is a system of learned behaviors, practiced by a group of people

   A. Cultural diversity

   B. Culture

   C. Bias

7. Positive responses to cultural diversity include which of the following

   A. Acceptance and knowledge

   B. Bias and knowledge

C. None of these

8. Which of the following are barriers to communication

A. Resident is difficult to understand

B. Advice is given

C. Resident cannot hear you

D. All of the above

9. All of the following are ways to make communication accurate except

A. Giving advice

B. Let some pauses happen

C. Ask for more

10. When helping residents, do not talk to other staff

A. True

B. False

11. A _____ is something that is definitely true

A. Opinion

B. Report

C. Fact

12. An _____ is something that is definitely true

A. Opinion

B. Report

C. Fact

13. Objective information is based on what you

A. See

B. Hear

C. Touch or smell

D. All of the above

14. _____ information is something you cannot or did not observe

   A. Objective

   B. Subjective

   C. Rejective

15. Inconsistence is

   A. Inability to control moving

   B. Inability to control the bladder or bowels

   C. Inability to control breathing

16. A resident shoes skin is pale or blue is called

   A. Edema

   B. Syncope

   C. Cyanotic

17. The root derm or derma means

   A. Head

   B. Neck

   C. Skin

18. The suffix " it is" means

   A. Incontinence

   B. Incision

   C. Complication

   D. Inflammation

19. _____ is an accident or unexpected event during the course of care

A. Incident

B. Impairment

C. Liability

Match the following

20. Hemiplegia_____   A. medical term for stroke

21. Hemiparesis _____   B. difficulty swallowing

22. Expressive aphasia _____   C. Inability to speak clearly

23. Receptive _____   D. inability to speak clearly

24. Dysphasia ___   E. weakness on one side of the body

25. Cerebrovascular accident (CVA) _____   F. Paralysis on one side the body

SECTION FIVE

1. _____ is term for measures practiced in healthcare facilities to prevent and control the spread of disease

    A. Medical asepsis

    B. Microbes

    C. Infection control

2. A _____ is a living thing or organism that is so small that it can be seen only through a microscope

    A. Virus

    B. Microorganism

    C. Infection

3. What is another name for microorganism

    A. Microbe

B. Amoeba

C. Bacteria

4. Infection occur when harmful microorganisms called pathogens invade the body and multiply

   True
   False
   None of the above

5. Which of the following infection is in the blood stream and is spread throughout the body

   A. Healthcare-associated infection

   B. Localized infection

   C. Systemic infection

6. A _____ is confined to a specific location in the body and has local symptoms

   A. Healthcare-associated infection

   B. Localized infection

   C. Systemic infection

7. _____ are infections that a patients acquire within healthcare settings that result from treatment for other conditions

A. Healthcare-associated infection

B. Localized infection

C. Systemic infection

8. _____ is the process of removing pathogens or the state of being free of pathogens

   A. Medical asepsis

   B. Surgical asepsis

   C. None of the above

9. What is the name given to the state of being free of al microorganisms not just pathogens

   A. Medical asepsis

B. Surgical asepsis

C. None of the above

10. The chain of infection is

   A. Is an uninfected person who could get sick

   B. Is a way of describing how disease is transmitted from one living being to another

   C. None of the above

11. Causative agents include which of the following

   A. Bacteria

   B. Viruses

   C. Fungi and protozoa

   D. All of the above

12. Examples of reservoirs include the

   A. Mouth

   B. Clothes

   C. Lungs, blood and the large intestine

13. The _____ is anybody opening on an infected person that allows pathogens to leave such as the nose, mouth, eyes or a cut in the skin

   A. Portal of entry

   B. Portal of exit

   C. None of the above

14. Which of the following describes how the pathogen travels from one person to the next person

   A. Mode of transmission

   B. Susceptible host

   C. None of the above

15. _____ is the condition that results from inadequate fluid in the body

    A. Infection

    B. Diarrhea

    C. Malnutrition

    D. Dehydration

16. Centers for Disease Control and prevention (CDC) is a governmental agency under the department of health and human services

    True
    False
    None of the above

17. Hand antisepsis refers to

    A. Hand-washing with either plain or antiseptic soap and water and using alcohol-based hand rubs

    B. Washing hands with water and soap or other detergents that contain an antiseptic agent

    C. None of the above

18. A _____ agent destroys or resists pathogen

    A. Microbes

    B. Microbial

    C. Antimicrobial

19. Personal protective equipment includes

    A. Gloves, gown

    B. Masks, goggles and face shields

    C. All of the above

20. _____ is a process that kills pathogens but not all microorganisms

    A. Disinfection

    B. Sterilization

C. Disposal

21. Which of the following are symptoms of hepatitis

    A. Chest pain

    B. Trouble breathing

    C. Mucus

    D. None of the above

22. Tuberculosis usually infect the

    A. Brain

    B. Lungs

    C. Heart

23. MRSA stands for

    A. Methicillin-resistant staphylococcus aureus

    B. Multidrug-resistant

    C. None of the above

24. _____ stands for vancomycin-resistant enterococcus

    A. HIV

    B. TB

    C. VRE

25. Which of the following is a spore forming bacteria which can be a part of the normal flora

    A. Enterococci

    B. Staphylococcus aureus

    C. Clostridium difficile

SECTION SIX

1. Which of the following includes our 5 senses

A. Sight and hearing

B. Touch and smell

C. Taste

D. All of the above

2. _____ is the loss of ability to move all or part of the body

A. Fracture

B. Paralysis

C. Sprain

3. It is very important to try to prevent accidents before they occur

A. True

B. False

4. A fracture is

A. A broken bone

B. A cracked bone

C. A severed bone

5. What fracture cause the greatest number of deaths and can lead to severe health problems

A. Shoulder

B. Leg

C. Hip

6. Which of the following factors raise the risk for falls except

A. Poor lighting

B. Shiny tiles

C. Slippery or wet floor

D. Throw rugs

7. _____ means confusion about person, place or time

   A. orientation

   B. disorientation

   C. identification

8. Never lock a wheel chair before transferring a resident into or out of it

   A. True

   B. False

9. What can be cause by dry heat

   A. Burns

   B. Cuts

   C. Scalds

10. Scalds are burns

A. True

B. False

11. _____ can occur when eating, drinking or swallowing medication

   A. Poisoning

   B. Gasping

   C. Slippery

   D. Choking

12. Residents must be sitting up straight when eating whether in a bed or a chair

   A. True

   B. False

13. An _____ is an injury that rubs off the surface of the skin

   A. Abrasion

B. Cut

C. Scratch

14. _____ means the process of burning

    A. Flammable

    B. Smoking

    C. Combustion

15. Which of the following requires that all hazardous chemicals must have a material safety data sheet

    A. MRSA

    B. HIV

    C. OSHA

16. Which of the following are examples of physical restraints

    A. Mitt restraints

    B. Belt restraints

    C. Side rails

    D. All of the above

17. _____ is death from a lack of air or oxygen

    A. Suffocation

    B. Atrophy

    C. Syncope

18. Understanding some basic principles of body mechanisms will help keep you and residents safe

    A. True

    B. False

19. _____ is the way the parts of the body with together whenever you move

A. Posture

B. Center of gravity

C. Body mechanics

20. Always try to catch a falling resident

A. true

B. false

21. Where does the center of gravity in your body point

    A. Where the most weight is concentrated

    B. Where the least weight is concentrated

    C. Where no weight is concentrated

22. The wider your support the more stable you are

    A. True

    B. False

23. A _____ moves an object by resting on a base of support

    A. Alignment

    B. Lever

    C. Counter of gravity

24. When you stand your weight is centered in your pelvis

    A. True

    B. False

25. Do not twist while you are moving an object

A. True

B. False

1. The first thing to do when you recognize a medical emergency is

   A. Turn on the AED

   B. Do nothing

   C. Assess the situation

   D. Start CPR

2. Which of the following means being mentally alert and having awareness of surroundings, sensations and thoughts

   A. Conscious

   B. Breathing

   C. Unconscious

   D. None of the above

3. Checking a person for injury include all of the following except

   A. Medical alert tags

   B. Nausea and vomiting

   C. Severe bleeding

   D. Changes in consciousness

4. _____ is an emergency care given immediately to an injured person

   A. CPR

   B. Abdominal thrust

   C. BLS

   D. First aid

5. To open the airway you should use the

A. Head tilt-chin lift

B. Chin lift head tilt

C. Both a and b

D. None of the above

6. When giving CPR the correct rate of chest compressions to breaths are

    A. 15 chest compressions to 1 rescue breaths

    B. 30 chest compressions to 2 rescue breaths

    C. 20 chest compressions to 1 rescue breaths

    D. 35 chest compressions to 2 rescue breaths

7. AED stands for

    A. Automatic external defibrillator

    B. Auto external defibrillator

    C. Automated externally defibrillator

    D. Automated external defibrillator

8. Adequate breathing should be detected no longer than _____ seconds

    A. 15

    B. 5

    C. 10

    D. 20

9. How could you tell when someone is choking

    A. He/she would put their hands to their throat and cough

    B. He/she would ask you to hit them on the back

    C. He/she would ask for a glass of water

    D. None of the above

10. The method of attempting to remove an object from the airway of someone who is choking is call

    A. Abdominal slaps

    B. Abdominal thrusts

    C. Depressions

    D. Compressions

11. What occur when organs and tissues in the body do not receive an adequate blood supply

    A. Choking

    B. Dyspnea

    C. Syncope

    D. Shock

12. Dyspnea means

    A. Difficulty breathing

    B. Difficulty smelling

    C. Painful breathing

    D. Both a and c

13. All of the following are signs and symptoms of MI except

    A. Nausea and vomiting

    B. Perspiration

    C. Blurred vision

    D. Cold and clammy skin

14. What is the medical term use for heart attack

    A. Myocardial Ischemia

    B. Myocardial infarction (MI)

    C. Myocardium infarction

D. None of the above

15. What should be done to control bleeding

   A. With gloves on and clean, thick sterile pad press down hard directly on the bleeding wound until help arrive

   B. Press down hard directly on the bleeding wound with bare hands until help arrive

   C. Maintain normal body temperature

   D. All of the above

16. Which of the following is used to treat accidental poisoning

   A. Epsom salts

   B. Ipecac syrup

   C. Activated charcoal

   D. All of the above

17. _____ degree burns involves all three layers of the skin

   A. First degree

   B. Second degree

   C. Third degree

   D. Total degree

18. What is the medical term for fainting

   A. BLS

   B. Syncope

   C. Myocardial ischemia

   D. Myocardial infarction

19. Insulin reaction is also called

   A. Hypoglycemia

B. Hypokalemia

C. Hyperglycemia

D. Hyperkalemia

20. _____ is caused by having too little insulin

   A. Hypoglycemia

   B. Hyperkalemia

   C. Diabetic ketoacidosis (DKA)/hyperglycemia

   D. None of the above

21. Which of the following is not a true statement about seizures

   A. Do not leave a person alone during a seizure

   B. Help the person get up slowly while having a seizure

   C. Do not give liquid or food

   D. Do not try to restrain the person

22. _____ is a warning sign of a CVA

   A. Myocardial ischemia

   B. Syncope

   C. Emesis

   D. Epilepsy

23. Transient ischemic attack (TIA) is also known as

   A. Mini stroke

   B. Semi stroke

   C. Bi-lateral stroke

   D. Tri lateral stroke

24. The act of ejecting stomach contents through the mouth is

A. Sputum

B. Mucus

C. Vomiting or emesis

D. None of the above

25. Disasters can include

A. Fire, flood

B. Earthquake, hurricane

C. Severe weather

D. All of the above

SECTION EIGHT

1. Which of the following is the correct order of Maslow's hierarchy of needs

A. Self-esteem, belongingness, self-actualization

B. Safety, physical needs, love and belongingness, security

C. Self-actualization, self-esteem, belongingness and security

D. Physical need, safety and security, love and belongingness, self-esteem and self-actualization

2. Considering a whole system such as a whole person rather than dividing the system up into parts

A. Holistic

B. Mental

C. Independence

D. None of the above

3. Which of the following is not a basic human physical need

A. Safety

B. Food and water

C. Getting an ipad

D. Comfort

4. A loss of independence can cause which of the following

A. Depression

B. Poor self- image

C. Feelings of being useless

D. All of the above

5. _____ means to touch or rub sexual organs in order to give oneself or another person sexual pleasure

A. Mensuration

B. Masturbation

C. Menstruation

D. Menopause

6. A person who has a desire for persons of the same sex is called a

A. Transsexual

B. Bisexual

C. Heterosexual

D. Gay

7. A woman whose sexual orientation is to women

A. Lesbian

B. Gay

C. Transsexual

D. Bisexual

8. Spirituality means

A. Relating to the spirit or soul

B. Relating to the mind

C. Relating to the way we conduct our selves

D. None of the above

Fill in the blank

Atheists   Buddhism   Christianity   Islam   Judaism   Islam

9. Believe that life is filled with suffering that caused by desire _____

10. Believe Jesus Christ was the son of God and that he died so their sins would be forgiven _____

11. Believe in reincarnation, karma and do not eat beef _____

12. Pray five times a day facing Mecca, the holy city for their religion _____

13. People who claim that there is no God _____

14. Do not do work from Friday sundown to Saturday sundown _____

15. Fasting means

A. Eating vegan food

B. Eating soul food

C. Not eating food or eating very little food

D. None of the above

16. _____ do not eat any animals or animal products such as eggs or dairy products

A. Vegetarian

B. Vegans

C. Ovo vegetarians

D. Lacto vegetarians

17. A highly contagious viral disease that strikes nearly all children is

A. Leukemia

B. SIDS

C. Ageism

D. Chicken pox

18. _____ is a maltreatment include not providing adequate food, clothing or support

  A. Child neglect

  B. Trauma

  C. Premature

  D. Disability

19. School-age children age from

  A. 12 to 18

  B. 3 to 6

  C. 6 to 12

  D. 18 to 40

20. _____ is a form of cancer

  A. Chicken pox

  B. Bulimia

  C. Leukemia

  D. SIDS

21. What is the study of health, wellness and disease later in life

  A. Gerontology

  B. Geriatrics

  C. Ageism

  D. Cognitive

22. The study of the aging process in people from mid-life through old age is called

A. Scientology

B. Geriatrics

C. Zoology

D. Gerontology

23. Prejudice towards stereotyping of against older persons or the elderly is called

A. Ageism

B. Anorexia

C. Old age

D. Gigantism

24. _____ refer to disabilities that are at birth or emerge during child-hood

A. Developmental disabilities

B. Down syndrome

C. Spina bifida

D. Cerebral palsy

25. Spina bifida literally means

A. Crack spine

B. Rip spine

C. Split spine

D. Age spine

SECTION NINE

1. What is the name for the condition in which all of the body's systems are working at their best

A. Homeostasis

B. Hormones

C. Glands

D. Digestion

2. The body is divided into _____ systems

A. 7

B. 9

C. 10

D. 11

3. Body systems are made up of

A. Cells

B. Glands

C. Tissues

D. Organs

4. What are the building block of our bodies

A. Organs

B. Cells

C. Tissues

D. Glands

5. Posterior or dorsal means

A. Away from the body

B. The back of the body or body part

C. The front of the body or body part

D. Closer to the torso

6. The largest organ and system in the body is the

A. Skin

B. Endocrine

C. Reproductive

D. Musculoskeletal

7. Normal changes of aging include which of the following

A. Skin is less elastic

B. Nails are harder and more brittle

C. Hair thins and may turn gray

D. All of the above

8. Which of the following is not a part of the skin

A. Epidermis

B. Dermis

C. Epicardium

D. Subcutaneous

9. How many bones the skeleton has

A. 206

B. 210

C. 220

D. 212

10. The point at where two bones meet is call a

A. Tissue

B. Contract

C. Glands

D. Joint

11. _____ provide movement of body parts to maintain posture and to produce heat

   A. Joint

   B. Muscles

   C. Cells

   D. Organs

12. Which of the following is not included in normal changes of aging

   A. Bone loss density

   B. Muscles weaken and lose tone

   C. Height is gradually lost

   D. Grow 6 inches taller

13. Which one of the following is the two main part of the nervous system

   A. Central nervous system (CNS)

   B. Peripheral nervous system

   C. A and B

   D. None of the above

14. The three main sections of the brain are

   A. Cerebrum

   B. Brainstem

   C. Cerebellum

   D. All of the above

15. The outer part of the eye is called

   A. Sclera

   B. Retina

   C. Iris

D. Cornea

16. Ear wax and hair in the ear protect the ear from

    A. Light

    B. Foreign objects

    C. Water

    D. None of the above

17. The heart is a

    A. Bone

    B. Organ

    C. Muscle

    D. Artery

18. The contracting phase of the heart is the

    A. Expiration

    B. Diastole

    C. Systole

    D. Inspiration

19. The resting phase of the heart is the

    A. Diastole

    B. Respiration

    C. Inspiration

    D. Expiration

20. Normal changes of aging include which of the following

    A. Voice weakens

    B. Lung capacity decreases

C. Lung strength decreases

D. All of the above

21. _____ is the process of expelling solid wastes made up of the waste products of food that are not absorbed into cells

A. Digestion

B. Ingestion

C. Absorption

D. Elimination

22. Fecal/anal incontinence is the

A. Inability to control the bowels

B. Inability to control urine

C. Inability to control drooling

D. Inability to control bleeding

23. The reproductive system allows human beings to _____

A. Multiply

B. Separate

C. Reproduce

D. None of the above

24. _____ protects against a particular disease that is invading the body at a given time

A. Acquired immunity

B. Specific immunity

C. Nonspecific immunity

D. Invading immunity

25. What is the name of the clear yellowish fluid that carries disease-fighting cells called lymphocytes

A. Sperm

B. Lymph

C. Gonads

D. None of the above

SECTION TEN

1. _____ means helping residents into positions that will be comfortable and healthy for them

    A. Positioning

    B. Homeostasis

    C. Holistic

2. In the _____ position the resident lies flat on his back

    A. Lateral

    B. Prone

    C. Supine

3. A person in the _____ position is lying on his or her back

    A. Prone

    B. Lateral

    C. Supine

4. A person lying in the _____ position is lying on his or her stomach

    A. Prone

    B. Sims

    C. Fowlers

5. A person lying in the _____ position is partially reclined

A. Prone

B. Sims

C. Fowlers

6. A draw sheet is a extra sheet placed on top of the bottom sheet

A. True

B. False

7. _____ is rubbing or friction that results from the skin moving one way and the bone underneath it remaining fixed or moving in the opposite direction

A. Shearing

B. Bearing

C. Shaving

8. Moving a resident as a unit, without disturbing alignment of the body is

A. Block rolling

B. Wood rolling

C. Log rolling

9. To _____means to sit up with the feet over the side of the bed for a moment to regain balance

A. Swing

B. Dangle

C. Shake

10. The science of designing equipment and work tasks to suit the workers abilities

A. Transfer board

B. Ergonomics

C. Gait belt

11. A _____ is a safety device used to transfer residents who are weak, unsteady or uncoordinated

    A. Transfer belt

    B. Gait belt

    C. Safety belt

12. Where should the gait belt be placed

    A. Around both legs of the resident

    B. Around the waist of resident over clothing

    C. On the wheel chair

13. What is the name of the equipment that can help transfer residents

    A. Transfer belt

    B. Gait belt

    C. Slide or transfer belt

14. A stretcher is another word for

    A. Cane

    B. Gurney

    C. Crutch

15. Which of the following equipment prevents wear and tear on your body

    A. Stretcher

    B. Mechanical or hydraulic lift

    C. Sling

16. Which of the following statements are not true about a mechanical lift

    A. You and the resident would not get hurt if you use the lift improperly

    B. You must be trained on the specific lift you will be using

C. Lifts help prevent injury to you and the resident

17. Which of the following statements are true about transferring a resident onto and off a toilet

   A. Position wheelchair at a right angle to toilet

   B. Ask resident to push against the arm rests of the wheelchair and stand

   C. All of the above

18. What is another word for walking

   A. Ambulation

   B. Pacing

   C. Moving

19. A resident who is ambulatory is

   A. One who can move in bed

   B. One who can get out of bed and walk

   C. None of the above

20. The purpose of a cane is to

   A. Help with balance

   B. Help visually impaired resident

   C. None of the above

21. The _____ cane is a straight cane with a curved handle at the top

   A. C cane

   B. Quad cane

   C. Functional grip cane

22. This type of cane has a grip handle rather than a curved handle

   A. C cane

   B. Quad cane

C. Functional grip cane

23. Which cane is designed to bear more weight than the other canes

    A. C cane

    B. Quad cane

    C. Functional grip cane

24. What equipment can be used when the resident can bear some weight on the legs

    A. Walker

    B. Cane

    C. Crutches

25. Residents who can bear no weight or limited weight on the leg use

    A. Walker

    B. Cane

    C. Crutches

SECTION ELEVEN

Fill in the blanks

Wants, them   time, condition   consciousness, confused   introduce, position
Friendly   formal   resident   arrives   bed, tidy   admission, kit   welcome, wanted   tour
valuables

1. Prepare the room before the resident _____

2. Make sure the _____ is made and the room is _____

3. A _____ _____ is usually in the patient room before he/she is admitted

4. When a new resident arrives at the facility note the _____ and _____

5. Observe the new resident for level of _____ and if he/she seems _____

6. _____ yourself and state your _____

7. Smile and be _____

8. Always call the person by his/her _____ name until they tell you what they want to be call

9. Never rush the new _____

10. Make sure the new resident feel _____ and _____

11. Offer to take the resident on a _____

12. Ask the new resident if he/she brought any _____

13. Place personal items where the resident _____ _____

True and False

14. Providing fresh water is something you should do every time you leave a resident's room

15. Report any changes in resident's weight to the nurse

16. Residents do not have the right to receive advance notice of any room or roommate change

17. Sphygmomanometer is used to measure blood pressure

18. Alcohol wipes cannot be used for infection and minor wound care

19. Otoscope is an instrument used to examine the eye

20. The dorsal recumbent position is used to examine the chest, breasts and abdomen

21. Lithotomy position is used to examine the rectum

22. To determine height on a standing scale gently lower the measuring rod until it rests flat on the resident's head

23. Admission kit will contain a urine specimen cup, personal care items, drinking glass, tooth paste and soap

24. Resident should not be told of their rights until after admission

25. The room should be prepare when the new resident arrives

SECTION TWELVE

True and false

1. Illness and disability cause great stress

2. Common noises in facilities can upset and irritate residents

3. Caffeinated drinks such as coffee or some teas do not prevent sleep, fatigue and irritability

4. A resident room is not his/her home and should not be treated with respect

5. Providing a clean, safe and orderly environment is an essential part of your job

6. Normally Beds are kept at their highest horizontal position

7. The water pitcher and cup are kept in the bedside stand drawer

8. It is important to always place the call light within the resident's reach

9. Curtains and screens block sounds from the other rooms

10. You do not have to wear gloves when rinsing bedpans and urinals

11. Sleep is a natural period of rest for the mind and body

12. The cadian rhythm is 24 hour day night cycle

13. Insomnia is the lack of ability to fall asleep or stay asleep

14. Sheets that are damp, wrinkled or bunched up under a resident is not uncomfortable

15. Hold soiled linen close to your body and place it in the proper container immediately

16. An occupied bed is a bed made while the resident is not in it

17. It is easier to make a bed when the resident is in it

18. Hospital corners help keep the flat sheet smooth under the resident

19. A close bed is a bed completely made with the bedspread and blankets in place

20. A surgical bed is made to accept residents who are returning to bed on stretchers or gurney

21. Good lighting is not important to residents

22. Always knock and wait to receive permission before entering

23. If resident seem sad, anxious, or fearful just ignore them

24. You do not have to keep a resident room neat and clean

25. An emesis basin is a kidney-shaped basin often used when giving mouth care

SECTION THIRTEEN

1. _____ is the term used to describe practices to keep our bodies clean and healthy

   A. Hygiene

   B. Grooming

   C. ADL

   D. None of the above

2. What is refer to as practices like caring for fingernails and hair

   A. Hygiene

   B. Grooming

   C. ADL

   D. None of the above

3. Which of the following is not included in a.m. care

   A. Offering a bedpan

   B. Giving a back rub

   C. Helping the resident to wash face and hands

   D. Assisting with mouth care before breakfast

4. _____ are areas of the body that bear much of its weight

   A. Pressure sores

   B. Bony prominences

   C. Pressure points

   D. None of the above

5. The areas of the body where the bone lies close to the skin is

A. Pressure sore

B. Pressure points

C. Hygiene

D. Bony prominences

6. A pressure sore is also call a

A. Decubitus ulcer

B. Pressure points

C. Broken skin

D. None of the above

7. How many stages of pressures are there

A. 2

B. 4

C. 3

D. 5

8. In what stage is the full skin loss with major destruction

A. Stage 1

B. Stage 2

C. Stage 4

D. Stage 3

9. In what stage is the skin intact but there is redness that is not relieved within 15 to 30 minutes

A. Stage 4

B. Stage 2

C. Stage 3

D. Stage 1

10. A _____ skin or _____ skin may be placed under the resident to absorb moisture

    A. Goat, pig

    B. Cow, dog

    C. Sheep, chamois

    D. None of the above

11. _____ heel protectors help keep feet properly aligned and prevent pressure sores

    A. Stuffed

    B. Padded

    C. Packed

    D. Shield

12. There are many types of ointments, creams and lotions that are used to treat, soften and protect the skin

    A. True

    B. False

    C. Maybe

    D. None of the above

13. _____ is a weakness of muscles in the feet and ankles that causes difficulty with the ability to flex the ankles and walk normally

    A. Foot pop

    B. Foot roll

    C. Foot curl

    D. Foot drop

14. What help prevent foot drop

A. Footboards

B. Foot stools

C. Foot roll

D. Foot curls

15. Hand rolls does not keep fingers from curling too tightly

A. True

B. False

C. Both of the above

D. None of the above

16. A _____ is a device such as a splint or brace that helps support and align a limb and improve its function

A. Splint device

B. Brace device

C. Orthotic device

D. Pillow device

17. The perineum is the

A. Vocal and skin area

B. Mucus and genital area

C. Genital and back area

D. Genital and anal area

18. A _____ is a substance added to another substance changing its effect

A. Additive

B. Subtractive

C. Partial

D. None of the above

19. Common sites for pressure sores are

    A. Thigh

    B. Shoulder

    C. Chest, nose and hands

    D. None of the above

20. The _____ is the are from the pubis to the upper thighs

    A. Buttock

    B. Groin

    C. Abdomen

    D. Perineal

21. A _____ is a sturdy chair designed to be placed in a bathtub or shower

    A. Geri chair

    B. Wheel chair

    C. Shower chair

    D. None of the above

22. Pediculosis is an

    A. Infestation of mice

    B. Infestation of pest

    C. Infestation of bugs

    D. Infestation of lice

23. _____ is an excessive shedding of dead skin cells from the scalp

    A. Scab

    B. Dandruff

C. Scratch

D. Crack

24. The medical term for bad breath is

   A. Edentulous

   B. Aspiration

   C. Halitosis

   D. Pediculosis

25. Edentulous means

   A. Having no teeth

   B. Having no sweat

   C. Having no pain

   D. Having bad breath

SECTION FOURTEEN

1. Which of the following is the normal temperature range for the oral method

   A. 96.6 - 98.6 degrees F

   B. 97.9 - 100.6 degrees F

   C. 97.6 - 99.6 degrees F

   D. 95.6 - 98.9 degrees F

2. Which of the following is the normal temperature range for the rectal method

   A. 98.6 - 100.6 degrees F

   B. 96.7 - 98.6 degrees F

   C. 95.6 – 98.9 degrees F

   D. 98.6 – 99.9 degrees F

3. Which of the following is another word for mouth

   A. Axillary

   B. Rectal

   C. Tympanic

   D. Oral

4. Which of the following is another word for ear

   A. Axillary

   B. Rectal

   C. Tympanic

   D. Oral

5. Oral thermometers are usually _____ in color

   A. Yellow

   B. Green or blue

   C. Black

   D. Lavender

6. Rectal thermometers are usually _____ in color

   A. Yellow

   B. Green

   C. Blue

   D. Red

7. Which temperature is considered to be the most accurate

   A. Rectal

   B. Oral

   C. Tympanic

D. Axillary

8. Which temperature is considered to be the least accurate

    A. Oral

    B. Tympanic

    C. Axillary

    D. Rectal

9. Why are mercury free thermometers safer than the mercury thermometers?

    A. They are more expensive than mercury thermometers

    B. They do not contain dangerous substance like mercury

    C. They are easier to read than mercury thermometers

    D. They are easier to hold

10. Where is the most common site for monitoring the pulse located

    A. In between the elbow and the shoulder

    B. In between the thigh and the leg

    C. On the feet

    D. On the inside of the wrist

11. Where is the brachial pulse located

    A. In between the elbow and the shoulder

    B. On the side of the neck

    C. On the feet

    D. On the left side of the chest

12. Which of the following is not a common pulse site

    A. Radial

    B. Apical

C. Femoral

D. All of the above

13. A _____ is an instrument designed to listen to sounds within the body

    A. Sphygmomanometer

    B. Stethoscope

    C. Pen

    D. Thermometer

14. What is the process of breathing air into the lungs

    A. Perspiration

    B. Dyspnea

    C. Respiration

    D. Expiring

15. Count the heart beat for _____ full minute to measure apical pulse

    A. 1

    B. 3

    C. 2

    D. 4

16. The normal respiration rate for adults ranges from

    A. 40 to 60

    B. 12 to 16

    C. 15 to 30

    D. 12 to 20

17. Infants normally breath at a rate of _____ to _____

    A. 24 to 30

B. 15 to 35

C. 30 to 40

D. 12 to 16

True and false

18. Heat relieves pain and muscular tension

19. Hot application can stop bleeding

20. Ice packs is consider to be a dry applicator

21. Disposable heat compresses are used more than once and then discarded

22. Sitz baths clean perineal wounds and reduce inflammation and pain

23. Sterile dressing do not cover open or drain wounds

24. IV stands for intravenous or into a vein

25. A nasal cannula is a piece of metal tubing that fits around the face

SECTION FIFTEEN

1. _____ is how the body uses food to maintain health

   A. Carbohydrates

   B. Nutrition

   C. Fats

   D. Protein

2. What is something found in food that provides energy, promote good health and helps regulate metabolism

   A. Protein

   B. Fat

   C. Vegetables

   D. Nutrient

3. _____ are part of every body cell

    A. Protein

    B. Grains

    C. Minerals

    D. Fruits

4. Carbohydrates can be divided into _____ basic types

    A. 4

    B. 2

    C. 3

    D. 1

5. Fats help the body store _____

    A. Vegetables

    B. Fruits

    C. Energy

    D. Milk

6. Vitamins _____,_____, _____ and _____ are fat-soluble vitamins

    A. A, D, E and K

    B. B, C and D

    C. K, B, and E

    D. None of the above

7. Which of the following is not an example of a mineral

    A. Zinc, iron

    B. Calcium

    C. Magnesium

D. Vitamin b

8. One- half to two-thirds of our body weight is

    A. Fat

    B. Water

    C. Food

    D. Blood

9. Calcium is used for building _____ and _____

    A. Hair and skin

    B. Fingers and toes

    C. Bones and teeth

    D. Nose and mouth

10. _____ are the major source of monounsaturated fats (MUFA)

    A. Oils

    B. Milk

    C. Beans

    D. Meat

True and false

11. Physical activity and nutrition work together for better health

12. Many elderly people take a variety of medications which can affect the way food smells and tastes

13. Thickened liquid include water and juice

14. Nasogastric tube are inserted in through the stomach

15. Nursing assistants are responsible for inserting and discontinuing tubes

16. Food likes and dislikes are influenced by what you eat as a child

17. The dietary department also makes diet cards

Match the following

18. Low sodium diet _____   A. Nothing by mouth

19. Dysphagia _____   B. Restricted protein

20. Vegetarians _____   C. clear juices, broth, gelatin and popsicles

21. High-potassium diets ___   D. Helps with constipation

22. NPO _____   E. Do not eat fish or poultry

23. Low-protein diet _____   F. No salt added

24. Liquid diet _____   G. Get food high in potassium (Banana, grapefruit)

25. High-residue diet _____ H. Difficulty swallowing

ANSWERS

SECTION ONE

1. A

2. C

3. A

4. True

5. A

6. C

7. B

8. B

9. C

10. B

11. A

12. C

13. A

14. True

15. False

16. B

17. C

18. True

19. B

20. B

SECTION TWO

1. J

2. I

3. H

4. G

5. F

6. E

7. D

8. C

9. B

10. A

11. A

12. True

13. B

14. H

15. G

16. F

17. E

18. D

19. C

20. B

21. A

22. D

23. True

24. A

25. D

26. C

27. B

28. A

29. F

30. E

SECTION THREE

1. C

2. A

3. True

4. B

5. B

6. D

7. B

8. C

9. M

10. L

11. K

12. J

13. I

14. H

15. G

16. F

17. E

18. D

19. C

20. A

21. B

22. C

23. C

24. B

25. True

SECTION FOUR

1. C

2. A

3. True

4. True

5. B

6. B

7. A

8. D

9. A

10. True

11. C

12. A

13. D

14. B

15. B

16. C

17. C

18. D

19. A

20. F

21. E

22. D

23. C

24. B

25. A

SECTION FIVE

1. C

2. B

3. A

4. True

5. C

6. B

7. A

8. A

9. B

10. B

11. D

12. C

13. B

14. A

15. D

16. True

17. B

18. C

19. C

20. A

21. D

22. B

23. A

24. C

25. C

SECTION SIX

1. D

2. B

3. True

4. A

5. C

6. B

7. B

8. False

9. A

10. True

11. D

12. True

13. A

14. C

15. C

16. D

17. A

18. True

19. C

20. False

21. A

22. True

23. B

24. True

25. True

SECTION SEVEN

1. C

2. A

3. B

4. D

5. A

6. B

7. D

8. C

9. A

10. B

11. D

12. D

13. C

14. B

15. A

16. D

17. C

18. B

19. A

20. C

21. B

22. D

23. A

24. C

25. D

SECTION EIGHT

1. D

2. A

3. C

4. D

5. B

6. D

7. A

8. A

9. Buddhism

10. Christianity

11. Hinduism

12. Islam

13. Atheists

14. Juduism

15. C

16. B

17. D

18. A

19. C

20. C

21. B

22. D

23. A

24. A

25. C

SECTION NINE

1. A

2. C

3. D

4. B

5. B

6. A

7. D

8. C

9. A

10. D

11. B

12. D

13. C

14. D

15. A

16. B

17. C

18. C

19. A

20. D

21. D

22. A

23. C

24. B

25. B

SECTION TEN

1. A

2. C

3. B

4. A

5. C

6. True

7. A

8. C

9. B

10. B

11. A

12. B

13. C

14. B

15. B

16. A

17. C

18. A

19. B

20. A

21. A

22. C

23. B

24. A

25. C

SECTION ELEVEN

1. Arrives

2. Bed, tidy

3. Admission kit

4. Time, condition

5. Consciousness, confused

6. Introduce, position

7. Friendly

8. Formal

9. Resident

10. Welcome, wanted

11. Tour

12. Valuables

13. Wants, them

14. True

15. True

16. False

17. True

18. False

19. False

20. True

21. False

22. True

23. True

24. False

25. False

SECTION TWELVE

1. True

2. True

3. False

4. False

5. True

6. False

7. False

8. True

9. False

10. False

11. True

12. True

13. True

14. False

15. False

16. False

17. False

18. True

19. True

20. True

21. False

22. True

23. False

24. False

25. True

SECTION THIRTEEN

1. A

2. B

3. B

4. C

5. D

6. A

7. B

8. C

9. D

10. C

11. B

12. A

13. D

14. A

15. B

16. C

17. D

18. A

19. D

20. B

21. C

22. D

23. B

24. C

25. A

SECTION FOURTEEN

1. C

2. A

3. D

4. C

5. B

6. D

7. A

8. C

9. B

10. D

11. A

12. D

13. B

14. C

15. A

16. D

17. C

18. True

19. False

20. True

21. False

22. True

23. False

24. True

25. False

SECTION FIFTEEN

1. B

2. D

3. A

4. B

5. C

6. A

7. D

8. B

9. C

10. A

11. True

12. True

13. False

14. False

15. False

16. True

17. True

18. F

19. H

20. E

21. G

22. A

23. B

24. C

25. D

GOOD LUCK IN YOUR EXAMS!!!

OTHER TITLES FROM THE SAME AUTHOR:

1. Work At Home Jobs For Nurses & Other Healthcare Professionals

2. Nurses' Romance Series

3. BLS for Healthcare Providers Student Manual

4. Patient Care Technician Exam Review Questions: PCT Test Prep

5. Accept Challenges

6. EKG Technician Study guide

7. EKG Test Prep

8. Phlebotomy Test Prep Vol 1, 2, & 3

9. The Home Health Aide Textbook

10. CNA Exam Prep Volume One & Two

And Many More Books

Visit www.janejohn-nwankwo.com

www.bookaspeakernow.com

www. Healthcarepracticetest.com

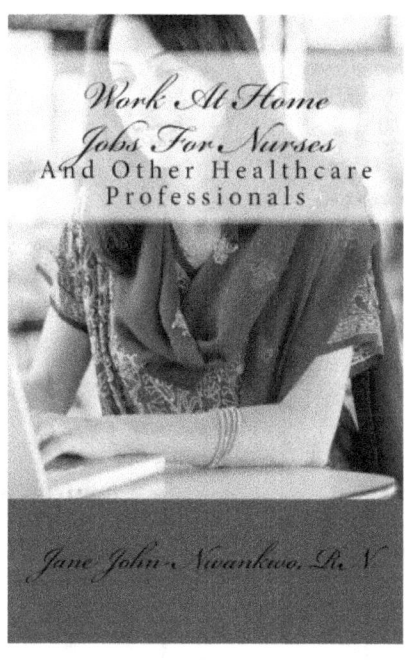

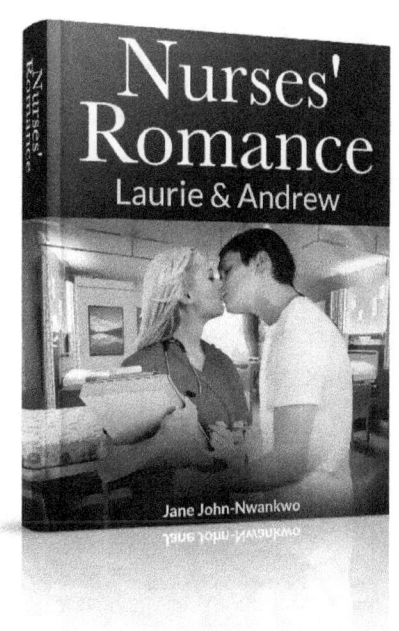

Search these books on amazon.com

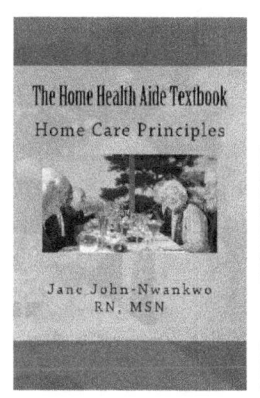

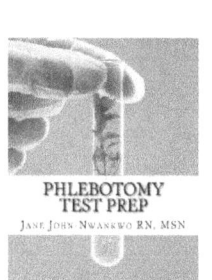

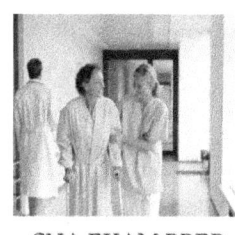

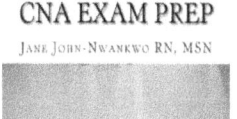

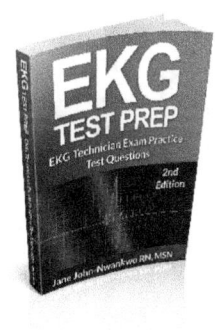

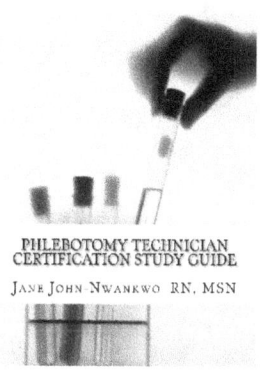

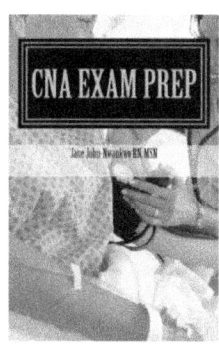

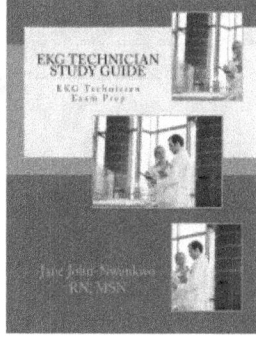

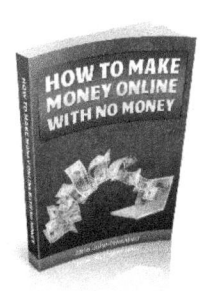

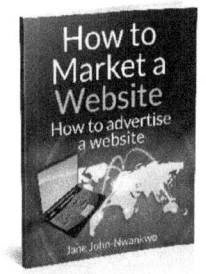

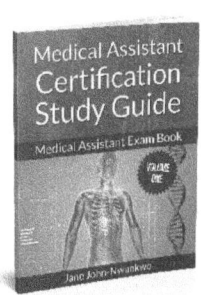

Search Jane John-Nwankwo on Amazon.com